How to Succeed in Nursing Assessments

How to Succeed in Nursing Assessments

Cariona Flaherty

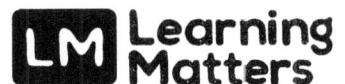

LM Learning Matters

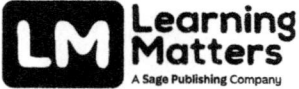

Learning Matters
A Sage Publishing Company

1 Oliver's Yard
55 City Road
London EC1Y 1SP

2455 Teller Road
Thousand Oaks
California 91320

10th Floor, Emaar Capital Tower 2
MG Road, Sikanderpur, Sector 26
Gurugram, Haryana – 122002
India

8 Marina View Suite 43-053
Asia Square Tower 1
Singapore 018960

Editor: Laura Walmsley
Assistant editor: Sahar Jamfar
Senior project editor: Chris Marke
Marketing manager: Ruslana Khatagova
Cover design: Bhairvi Vyas
Typeset by: C&M Digitals (P) Ltd, Chennai, India

Library of Congress Control Number: 2025943865

British Library Cataloguing in Publication Data

A catalogue record for this book is available from the
British Library

ISBN 978-1-5296-8502-2
ISBN 978-1-5296-8505-3 (pbk)

Contents

Acknowledgements

The authors would like to acknowledge the support and kindness shown by editorial team Ruth Lilly and Martha Cunneen.

About the author

Cariona Flaherty, RGN, Higher Dip, BSc (Hons), PGCHE, SFHEA, is an Associate Professor and Head of School of Nursing and Midwifery (Interim) and NMC Correspondent at Middlesex University. Cariona is a specialist critical care nurse with extensive experience in both senior clinical roles and academic leadership. Drawing on a strong clinical foundation, she currently leads nursing and midwifery education strategy at Middlesex University. Her role also involves close collaboration with external partners, further education institutions and accreditation bodies. Passionate about assessment literacy and student success, Cariona adopts a compassionate leadership approach to support students in achieving their potential. Her research interests focus on critical thinking in nurse education and pedagogical practices that foster inclusive and enriching learning environments.

About the contributor

Dr Phil Barter is the Academic Director of Middlesex University Mauritius, where he leads the academic vision and strategic development of the campus. With a strong background in higher education leadership, Dr Barter is committed to fostering academic excellence, innovation in teaching, learning and assessment in a student-centred approach. He has a wealth of experience in authentic assessment, curriculum development, quality assurance and international education, ensuring that Middlesex Mauritius continues to deliver a globally relevant and locally impactful education. Passionate about empowering both students and staff, Dr Barter champions inclusive practices and collaborative authentic learning environments that prepare students to graduate for success in a rapidly evolving world.

Introduction

Who is the book for?

This book is designing specifically for a diverse audience involved in the education and development of nurses. It is intended primarily for student nurses who are undertaking their training. This book can also serve as a valuable resource for educators who play a key role in guiding and preparing students who are looking to begin their nursing studies at university, as well as those who are teaching students who are already enrolled on nursing programmes. The content of the book links theory to practice by providing an overview of assessments and how they are linked to practice requirements, such as communication and written record keeping.

About the book

Nurse education is continuously evolving to meet the needs of the rapidly changing NHS and increasingly diverse patient demographics. As a result, students must be well prepared not only academically, but also practically to ensure they are prepared for practice.

While assessment traditionally has been seen as a way to test knowledge, there is a growing move towards making nursing assessments more authentic and reflective of clinical practice. This move presents a real opportunity for student nurses to engage more deeply with the practical aspects of assessment preparation which can, in turn, support practice. For example, using evidence to support your academic writing reflects the professional expectation to deliver evidence-based care in clinical practice. By learning how to critically appraise and apply research in assessments, students are also developing the analytical skills required for safe and effective patient care. In this way assessments should not be viewed as a barrier, but more of a tool of learning to think and act like a qualified nurse.

However, despite the potential benefits, the learning process involved in preparing and undertaking assessments is often overshadowed by the stress and anxiety associated with achieving a pass grade. Therefore, supporting students in understanding and engaging with assessment literacy as an opportunity for professional growth can play a crucial role in students' success with assessments.

This book was written with the aim of making assessments easier for students to understand, offering simple and practical guidance on how to approach any type of assessment throughout your nursing programme. Although the level of detail provided in this book derives from a simple and practical approach, the advice given can be applied as assessment increases in complexity.

Book structure

Chapter 1: Assessment literacy and authentic assessment in nursing. This chapter begins with an overview of what is meant by the term 'assessment literacy' in nursing assessments. It provides an introduction into the various types of assessments and outlines the principles of authentic assessment. In undertaking any assessment you will need to know how to interpret the assessment brief and understand the marking criteria – this chapter supports this and provides some practical tips.

Chapter 2: Written assessments. Written assessments are a common feature across nurse education and provide a wealth of opportunity for students to develop a range of communication, reading and analytical skills which are underpinned by evidence. This chapter provides an overview of written assessments, focusing on essays that include reflection. The purpose of this chapter is not to teach you about reflection, but instead to introduce you to reflective models used to support reflective writing.

Chapter 3: Presentations. These can be quite daunting for students, but continue to be used in various formats such as individual, group, live or narrated. This chapter provides practical advice on how to plan and deliver a live or narrated presentation, individually or as part of a group. There is a wider discussion on group presentations, including the benefits and challenges of working as part of a team, and how teamwork reflects the role of a qualified nurse.

Chapter 4: Quality improvement. Quality improvement is a drive across the NHS and wider care sector aimed at improving care throughout data driver improvement projects involving key stakeholders such as patients and their families. This type of assessment is often seen in nurse education where a student assessment may include writing a quality improvement proposal that reflects their practice experience. This chapter introduces quality improvement and outlines how to undertake a quality improvement project as an assessment within nursing.

Chapter 5: Dissertation (literature review). Understanding how to use, read, collect and interpret literature is an important feature within student nurse assessments. This is crucial learning to support the delivery of informed practice and research-driven patient care. This chapter introduces the concept of a dissertation with a focus on undertaking a literature review. The learning from this chapter can be applied across all chapters because using the literature is applicable to all student nursing assessments.

Chapter 6: Observed structured clinical examination (OSCE). Demonstrating your ability to apply learning to practice is fundamental and not only assessment in clinical practice. An OSCE is a form of assessment where you will undertake the assessment and management of a fictious patient. This chapter provides an overview of the components of an OSCE assessment and discusses the importance and relevance of this type of assessment within nurse education.

Chapter 7: Simulation and virtual reality. Simulation and simulated practice learning continue to be widely integrated into nurse education and this type of learning has several benefits, including the developing of digital literacy among nursing students. Simulation and virtual reality offer students the opportunity to learn in a safe and supportive environment that reflects clinical practice. This chapter addresses the role of simulation within nurse education and gives practical ways to prepare for simulation-based assessments.

Chapter 8: Written exams: drug calculation. Written exams assess a range of knowledge and are employed within nurse education to access a student's ability to apply learning to practice, think critically and link theory to practice. The assessment for drug calculations is underpinned by the Nursing and Midwifery Council (NMC, 2018) and this is assessed via an exam with a 100 per cent pass grade required. This chapter discusses the purpose of exams in nurse education, the various types of exams and some practical tips on how to prepare and succeed.

Learning features

This book incorporates learning features throughout the chapter to help guide your understanding and provide further learning for you. The goal is not to dilute learning, but to provide an accessible starting point for understanding assessments – encouraging you to see assessments as a positive opportunity to learn and demonstrate what you know. The learning features include:

1. *case studies*, used throughout to reflect the student experience when facing challenges in preparing for and completing various assessments. Each case study includes questions designed to support and deepen your thinking and learning. Case studies are typically presented at the beginning of each chapter; however, in some chapters, they are included throughout to illustrate a student's thinking as their learning increases in complexity.
2. *activities*, included in each chapter to provide further learning. These activities may ask you to reflect on your experience, or to think critically about an area of assessment. The activities provide you with the opportunity to pause and think about the learning that each section within the chapters has provided. Model answers are provided at the end of each chapter to further enhance your learning.
3. *annotated further reading*, provided at the end of each chapter. The list is not exhaustive and there is a broad selection of journals, books, web links and videos provided to support your further reading.

Each chapter provides links to the other chapters where required and asks you to refer to previous chapters to further your learning. You can work through the book using a linear approach, or dip in and out of each chapter as you need it.

We hope you enjoy this book and that it provides a practical and easy-to-use guide to support you undertaking your assessment. We wish you all the best of luck with your assessments.

References

Nursing and Midwifery Council (NMC) (2018) *The Code: Professional Standards of Practice and Behaviour for Nurses, Midwives and Nursing Associates*. London: NMC.

Chapter 1

Assessment literacy and authentic assessment in nursing

Dr Phil Barter

Chapter aims

By the end of this chapter, you should be able to:

- explain what assessment literacy is in the context of nursing;
- identify the different types of assessment you will encounter;
- explain what is meant by the term 'authentic assessment';
- understand how assessment may change throughout your degree programme;
- learn how your assessments are marked.

Introduction

Well done on starting your nursing degree programme; I am sure this is an important step for you. One of the most important words to you in the next few years of study is *assessment*. I am sure that there will be times where it is the last word you want to hear, but there will also be times where hearing that gives you joy and a sense of achievement. In this chapter we're talking about assessment in relation to your nursing programme, but what is assessment? Why is assessment an important thing for you to understand and be literate about? Assessment is simply the way you have an opportunity to demonstrate your knowledge and understanding of a given task. Typically, assessments in the context of your degree programme run over a year, as a continuous form, or as a singular, more summative assessment at the end of a period of learning. The assessments you undertake will generate a set of grades which will inform the final classification of degree you will be awarded. So the importance of assessment in any form cannot be underestimated (Koretsky et al., 2022).

A simple understanding of how an assessment is completed will enhance your chance of success on your nursing programme. In the ever-changing world of education it's important for you to understand the evolving assessment landscape, so that you are prepared for any future changes which might occur during your nursing degree programme. For example, a simple presentation may now be given the brief of being digital, which simply means you are being asked to present in a variety of ways. This will ensure you meet the needs of future employment and the skills required in nursing. In recent years, universities and academics have reviewed assessment and how it helps prepare students for the workplace. The review has meant a move towards using the term 'authentic assessments', which means your assessment will align which what you do in practice – for example, drug calculations for nursing. This chapter will begin with an overview of the terms 'assessment', 'assessment literacy' and 'authentic assessment'. A brief introduction to the different types of assessment will be provided, followed by an overview of how your assessment may be marked. The chapter will provide activities that you can work through to support your learning.

Assessment

Assessments are designed to measure your progress and ensure you have acquired the necessary skills and knowledge required for your field. They can take many forms, such as exams, essays, practical tasks and projects. Each type of assessment has its own set of criteria and methods of evaluation. Understanding these different types of assessments and their purposes will help you approach them with confidence and clarity. By developing your assessment literacy you can better navigate the academic requirements of your programme and, ultimately, succeed in your studies. Now let's take a look at what is meant by the term 'assessment literacy'.

Assessment literacy

Throughout this book, we'll be referring to *assessment literacy*. This simply means an understanding of the different types of assessments you might be asked to complete, such as formative assessments, which provide ongoing feedback, and summative assessments, which evaluate your cumulative knowledge. Gaining this understanding will enable you to interpret tasks clearly and structure your assessments appropriately. Knowing what an assessment is asking you to do in relation to its modality will also help you understand how it will be marked. These elements form part of your overall assessment literacy, making you better informed to meet the requirements and demonstrate your knowledge and skills in an appropriate manner (Price, 2012; Levi and Inbar-Lourie, 2020). Having looked at assessment literacy, let's move on to *authentic assessment*.

Authentic assessment

An assessment is deemed to be authentic if it prepares you for tasks that you will undertake as a qualified nurse. Traditionally, assessments might have been in the form of essays and exams to evaluate your knowledge on any given module as part of a programme. Authentic assessment would be in the form of an observed structured clinical examination (OSCE), or by producing a report or a digital presentation. These assessments evaluate the same fundamental knowledge and skill required to complete your programme, but they ask you to present this knowledge in a format more likely to be encountered in employment. In other words, an authentic assessment reflects practice. Throughout your nursing programme, the level of authenticity in assessments typically increases as you progress. In the first year, you might only get a taste of authentic, practical examinations, with most assessments being traditional in nature. As you move through the subsequent years in a typical three-year degree, the balance between traditional and authentic assessments will shift, with a greater emphasis on authenticity. Throughout this chapter, we'll identify the different assessments and what they mean, as well as improve your understanding of what is meant by authenticity in these assessment modalities (Ajjawi et al., 2020). This holistic approach to assessments will help you build a strong foundation of knowledge and skills that are directly applicable to your chosen field, enhancing your employability and readiness for the challenges that lie ahead as a practising nurse (Poindexter et al., 2015; Quinlan et al., 2024).

Activity 1.1 Reflection

Using the table below, try and match the key terms with the appropriate definition.

Table 1.1 Key terms

Term		Definition	
1	Assessment	A	The level to which the assessments are appropriate for real-world practice or workplace settings
2	Authentic assessment	B	An understanding of the different types of assessments
3	Assessment literacy	C	An understanding of how to demonstrate your knowledge and skills appropriately in an assessment and its relevance to the workplace or practice setting
4	Authentic assessment literacy	D	An opportunity to demonstrate your knowledge and understanding in a set task

A model answer is provided at the end of this chapter.

Why is authentic assessment important?

By engaging with authentic assessments, you can develop competencies that are directly relevant to your field. These assessments simulate real-world scenarios, allowing you to apply theoretical knowledge to practical problems. This process enhances your critical thinking, problem-solving abilities and overall readiness for professional challenges. Furthermore, authentic assessments often require you to collaborate with others, improving your communication and teamwork skills, which are essential in most professional environments.

The transition from academic settings to professional life can be daunting, but authentic assessments help bridge this gap. They provide a preview of what to expect in your future career, allowing you to build confidence and adapt to professional expectations gradually. This preparation is invaluable, as it equips you with the tools and mindset needed to thrive in your chosen career path (Wiewiora and Kowalkiewicz, 2019).

Below is a quick task to help you build an understanding of the difference between authentic assessments and traditional assessments. This exercise will highlight how authentic assessments can help you develop your skills throughout your studies and prepare you for employment. Engaging with this task will give you insights into the practical applications of your academic learning and how it translates to real-world job performance (Poindexter et al., 2015; Quinlan et al., 2024).

Activity 1.2   Critical thinking

1. From the list of assessment tasks below, can you correctly identity which ones are authentic assessments and which are non-authentic assessments?
2. As an extra task can you classify any assessment task from your own degree programme?

Table 1.2   Authentic and non-authentic

	Task	Authentic or non-authentic
1	Complete an essay explaining the difference between pre-2021 and post-2021 hand hygiene guidelines	
2	Review the patient's records and administer the correct dosage of medication	
3	Using PowerPoint™ present your patient's case file	
4	Demonstrate how to take blood pressure on a mannequin	
5	Complete a scientific investigation into the absorption rates of different blood types and present your findings in a lab report format	
6	Complete a critical review on the different manual handling protocols	
7	Complete a practical scenario where a patient has collapsed	
8	Three-hour unseen exam paper on human anatomy	
9	Essay question: how do you measure heart rate and blood pressure accurately?	
10	Demonstrate how to safely turn a patient	

A model answer is provided at the end of this chapter.

Types of assessment

Written assessment

A *written assignment* is generally a non-authentic form of assessment. Generally speaking, this type of assignment will have an assignment brief which will be given to you or available for you to download. The assignment brief will normally outline the structure as an introduction, a middle part and then a concluding section. There will also be a list of resources or reading to help you complete the assignment; your lecturers will provide this. Typical examples of this type of assessment are essays, case study reports and lab reports (Price, 2012; Levi and Inbar-Lourie, 2020). Written assessment will be looked at further in Chapter 2.

Narrated and oral presentations

Narrated presentations and *oral presentations* are similar and, fundamentally, they ask you to demonstrate your understanding of knowledge in a non-written format. A narrated presentation typically will be a PowerPoint slide or poster, with you verbally explaining the points to demonstrate depth of your understanding. Normally, oral presentations would require you to physically present a poster or presentation and involve answering any questions that are asked by the assessors (normally your lecturers). As previously mentioned, the marks awarded for presentations vary depending on whether you are presenting a poster or a presentation (Price, 2012; Levi and Inbar-Lourie, 2020). Presentations will be looked at further in Chapter 3.

Quality improvement project

A *quality improvement project* can be seen as an application of what you traditionally might have covered in a thesis or dissertation. You will be given a problem and be expected to articulate how you will evaluate and improve that problem. The format of this type of assessment is normally given out in an assignment brief which you might find in your module handbook. Typically, a quality improvement project needs to have the following sections:

- analysis to identify the problem;
- researched action plan outlining how you plan to solve the problem;
- evaluation to assess the effectiveness of your proposed action plan.

Quality improvement will be looked at further in Chapter 4.

Dissertation (literature review)

A *dissertation* or literature review can take different forms. For example, in more scientific and less practical subjects, a dissertation would be an outline of an area for investigation through experimental means with primary data collection normally taking place in a laboratory; whereas, for a dissertation in nursing collecting primary data would be difficult, therefore a literature review would be a more common approach. With a literature review-based dissertation, you would be asked to complete what's called *desktop research* where you have a subject or specific research question and you look at the literature to answer the question. For example, a dissertation may include the following sections:

- a research question will usually be at the start of your dissertation, and this is the main question you are trying to answer with your research;
- the literature review:
  - discusses the key texts and research that enable you to answer the research question
  - investigates in detail the subject in order to answer your research question;
- the methodological section:
  - you identify how you are going to investigate the identified research question
  - what research methods or practical studies you are going to undertake;
- the results and findings section:
  - you will analyse your results
  - give an indication of whether you've answered the research question;
- some dissertations would then also conclude with a small section on how your research findings can be applied to practice (Price, 2012; Levi and Inbar-Lourie, 2020).

Dissertations will be looked at further in Chapter 5.

OSCE

An OSCE is a form of assessment designed to evaluate your ability to apply knowledge in decision-making scenarios while also demonstrating practical clinical skills. It is seen as an opportunity for you to demonstrate your clinical competency in communication, note-taking, physical examination, clinical reasoning and medical knowledge, while also showcasing your ability to integrate these skills. This type of assessment is very common in nursing programmes as it allows you to demonstrate the required competencies for placement (Price, 2012; Levi and Inbar-Lourie, 2020). OSCEs will be looked at further in Chapter 6.

Simulation/VR

Simulation or *virtual reality* (VR) assessments are relatively new in higher education, but, similar to an OSCE, they allow you to practise your skills in a safe setting. Through the use of VR, the assessment environment can be adapted to see how your thinking develops through various situations and how you adjust to potentially taking a wrong turn and what corrective decisions you might make. The advantage of a VR simulation over an OSCE is that you can have multiple routes through the situation which allows you to then test your knowledge in different ways – rather than with the OSCE, which is often a set approach. VR and simulation are also great ways to test your practical skills in preparation for placement (Price, 2012; Levi and Inbar-Lourie, 2020). Simulation/VR will be looked at later in Chapter 7.

Written exams: drug calculation

Written exams are often seen as very traditional – even out-of-date – in some courses of higher education. However, there is a place for the written exam in some subjects. In nursing and health studies, written exams are mainly centred around the level of knowledge that you definitely need to have prior to entering practice and/or placement. Typically, this will be through a drug calculation exam where you are required to achieve 100 per cent pass mark (NMC, 2018). The format of these exams can vary by university, from being in a traditional examination hall with everyone completing a written paper to online through the use of a detailed multiple-choice question (MCQ) exam – or some combination of the two. Fundamentally, however, exams are testing your ability to recall information in a timed scenario for a particular purpose of meeting certain competencies (Price, 2012; Levi and Inbar-Lourie, 2020). Written exams will be looked at later in Chapter 8.

Activity 1.3   Reflection

Reflecting on any tasks you have completed on your degree to date and the sections above:

1. how were those assessments authentic?
2. how do you think the assessment could become more authentic and relevant to your nursing practice in the future?

As this is a reflection no model answer is provided.

How will your assessment be marked?

In this chapter so far, we have discussed different types of assessment, how assessment can be authentic and why that's important. The final part is to look at the two distinct types of assessment and how they will be marked (Price, 2012; Levi and Inbar-Lourie, 2020).

Formative assessment

Formative assessment is generally a practice assessment, designed to help you develop ideas for the submission of your final assessment. A formative assessment will often be shorter in length than the final or summative version of the assessment and the feedback will be more detailed and descriptive, giving you guidance towards creating an improved final assessment. The formative assessment will not have a grade associated with it, but the tone and the language of the feedback given should be something that you should carefully consider, as this will give you an indication of the current grade boundary your work sits in.

Summative assessment

A *summative* assessment will be a piece of work or exam at the end point of a module and will build on the work covered in the formative assessment. This submission will be marked in accordance with the marking criteria and/or rubric. The marking will lead to an overall summary comment about the work, identifying where it meets or fails to meet the criteria. The marking will also include a definite grade which will go towards your final module grade.

Marking and grading assessments

Your work will be marked generally in accordance with a grading criteria. The criteria might have several sections based around the structure of the assessment or be a more general outline of what the tutor is expecting. For example, if the assessment takes the form of an essay the criteria might include an introduction, middle section, conclusion and references. Alternately, there might be more specific sections included in the criteria such as sections around sources, presentation, formatting in general and writing style. Each of those criteria should be outlined for you prior to submitting the work and will usually have a percentage weighting or percentage of the mark going towards your final assignment. When you are completing your assignments, make sure you refer to the grading criteria; don't overlook easy marks like correct referencing, formatting and avoiding grammatical errors. These can boost your base mark above the pass level. Focus on understanding the tutor's criteria, developing coherent arguments and using subsections to structure your work. For presentations, follow format rules and use diagrams and images effectively. This guidance should be part of the assignment brief you receive; if not, ask your tutor for guidance.

   Using marking criteria and understanding how you can gain easier marks is important as this will contribute to the overall grade you receive. Grading often uses a rubric, which can help you see where you scored well and where you need to improve. Rubrics are useful for assessments as they show the difference between lower-, middle- and higher-grade marks. With the summative submission, you will typically receive an overall comment linked to the grading criteria and/or a rubric which will highlight exactly in which areas you've scored well or not so well. Now let's take a look at example marking criteria.

Activity 1.4   Critical thinking

Using the example marking criteria in Table 1.3, match the segments from assessment feedback and try to produce a grade to match the feedback.

Tables 1.3   Marking criteria

Criteria	70%+	60–9%	50–9%	40–9%	Less than 40%
Content: Topic chosen relevant and informative, with a depth of knowledge and understanding	Excellent and well-informed understanding of theories and concepts involved with topic	Good understanding of theories and concepts involved with topic	Demonstrate satisfactory knowledge and understanding of topic's theories and concepts	Adequate content, and limited depth of knowledge and understanding	Inadequate content and limited depth of knowledge and understanding
Communication: Interesting, relevant language, explanation of terminology	Very well expressed and very good understanding of content	Very well expressed; good understanding of content	Well expressed; understanding of content	Unclear expression of information; little understanding of content	Unclear and confusing; lack of understanding of content
References: Reference to sources, including directions for further study	Broad and relevant readings examined and used selectively in presentation	Good range of appropriate references used during the presentation	Conventional references and readings used within presentation	Adequate but limited use of references during presentation	Critique relies on some or one reference; evidence of unexamined personal opinion

Table 1.4   Marking criteria example

Example	Feedback	Grade
1	You set out your context and gave some clear outline of your presentation, which was a good starting point. However, you did not give a clear indication of what the technology was that you were going to implement, the presentation lacked details and your argument was confusing in places	
	In terms of areas for improvement, the references used in some sections to add depth to your understanding could have been more current in places and, in general, you needed more references in your presentation – three does not indicate the required level of reading for this master's-level piece of work	
	You cover the limitations and future areas of the implementation briefly, with some interesting points in general; it could be improved further by the use of references to support your approach	

Example	Feedback	Grade
2	Well done for producing this presentation; you use the technology to a reasonable standard to record your PowerPoint presentation. Your approach was clear and you spoke in depth about your chosen subject. The rationale for the implementation of the drug was good, but could do with strengthening to fully explain the thinking behind its use and linked with research where appropriate. Your analysis of references gave a good indication of your level of understanding of the topic. For the evaluation of the drug implementation, I would have liked to have seen some more specific methods based on research	
3	Well done for producing this presentation; you use the technology to a sound standard to record your presentation, with a good colour scheme and clear text	
	You set out your context and gave a clear outline of your presentation which was a good starting point to explain your implementation of your chosen handling method	
	In terms of areas for improvement, the references cited at the end of the presentation are extensive and very impressive, but these needed to be more readily cited throughout the slides	
	You cover the limitations and future areas of the implementation briefly, with some interesting points around the use of this method, which gave some good insight to your excellent understanding. Your evaluation again was clear, but it could be improved further by the use of references to support your approach	
4	Well done for producing this presentation; the production level is of the highest quality and you have shown expert skills in terms of utilising technology to produce this work. I really liked the way you embedded a video into the presentation to show the CPR method	
	Your implementation approach is clearly outlined and linked with research to support your choice of method	
	The rationale for the implementation of methods is strong and well planned, again linked with research where appropriate	
	The depth shown in your implementation and evaluation of the impact of the use of the chosen method is excellent; the only area for improvement would be to try to use more references	

The grade answers with explanations are provided at the end of this chapter.

Tips for working on your authentic assessment

This section will outline some tips for you to consider when completing your authentic assessments, which if applied should help you in being more successful in your assessments and, in turn, across the whole of your nursing programme.

1. **Use your placement knowledge:** one of the ways that you can maximise your opportunity to succeed in authentic assessment is using the knowledge gained on placement – because the nature of authentic assessment tasks is that they should relate to the skills in scenarios you have practised and completed during your placement hours.

2. **Use practical knowledge to support your academic work**: when you are completing an authentic assessment it might help you to position that task within the placement setting in your thoughts and think about how you would have completed it if you were in practice. So, in essence, the placement experience will give you the basis for your answer and then you use your academic skills to support this with literature and sources, making sure you reference appropriately.

3. **Keep a reflection diary**: after each shift during your placement, try to reflect on key knowledge points you've learned and write these down. Link these points to your academic modules. Building detailed notes to use in assessments will help you connect practical experience with theoretical knowledge. You will then be able to review the diary and link to a particular scenario, giving you an example you can use to help bridge knowledge and practice in your authentic assessment.

4. **Make good notes during theory sessions**: make notes during theory sessions to identify key information for your placement. This helps you recall useful knowledge for specific shifts and apply it effectively when you are on placement. Regular note-taking before theory and practical sessions enhances your understanding and will help you develop essential authentic skills for your practical competencies.

Conclusion

Assessments are a vital part of any educational programme; they evaluate your knowledge, skills and competencies and are crucial for academic success and professional readiness as a nurse. This chapter covered assessment literacy and authenticity, emphasising the importance of understanding assessment types and effective communication to be able to demonstrate your understanding in the appropriate format. Authentic assessment is vital for future employability, especially in health-related fields like nursing. Linking practice to theory can improve assignment outcomes; applying the principles discussed in this chapter should prepare you to meet the challenges of your academic journey and professional challenges. Chapter 2 will focus on written assessments, offering strategies for success.

Brief outline answers

Activity 1.1 Reflection

1	D
2	A
3	B
4	C

Activity 1.2 Critical thinking

	Task	Authentic or non-authentic
1	Complete an essay explaining the difference between pre-2021 and post-2021 hand hygiene guidelines	Non-authentic
2	Review the patient's records and administer the correct dosage of medication	Authentic

	Task	Authentic or non-authentic
3	Using PowerPoint™ present your patient's case file	Non-authentic
4	Demonstrate how to take blood pressure on a mannequin	Authentic
5	Complete a scientific investigation into the absorption rates of different blood types and present your findings in a lab report format	Authentic
6	Complete a critical review on the different manual handling protocols	Non-authentic
7	Complete a practical scenario where a patient has collapsed	Authentic
8	Three-hour unseen exam paper on human anatomy	Non-authentic
9	Essay question: how do you measure heart rate and blood pressure accurately?	Non-authentic
10	Demonstrate how to safely turn a patient	Authentic

Activity 1.4 Critical thinking

Example	Feedback	Grade	Explanation
1	You set out your context and gave some clear outline of your presentation, which was a good starting point. However, you did not give a clear indication of what the technology was that you were going to implement, the presentation lacked details and your argument was confusing in places In terms of areas for improvement, the references used in some sections to add depth to your understanding could have been more current in places and, in general, you needed more references in your presentation – three does not indicate the required level of reading for this master's-level piece of work You cover the limitations and future areas of the implementation briefly, with some interesting points in general; it could be improved further by the use of references to support your approach	Less than 40%	Lack of references Sound level of knowledge Confused argument
2	Well done for producing this presentation; you use the technology to a reasonable standard to record your PowerPoint presentation. Your approach was clear and you spoke in depth about your chosen subject. The rationale for the implementation of the drug was good, but could do with strengthening to fully explain the thinking behind its use and linked with research where appropriate. Your analysis of references gave a good indication of your level of understanding of the topic. For the evaluation of the drug implementation, I would have liked to have seen some more specific methods based on research	50+	Clear context Good rationale, but needed to be stronger Needed more references Needed more specific evaluation
3	Well done for producing this presentation; you use the technology to a sound standard to record your presentation, with a good colour scheme and clear text	60+	Clear context Good rationale

(Continued)

(Continued)

Example	Feedback	Grade	Explanation
	You set out your context and gave a clear outline of your presentation which was a good starting point to explain your implementation of your chosen handling method		Good range of references, but needed to use them more
	In terms of areas for improvement, the references cited at the end of the presentation are extensive and very impressive, but these needed to be more readily cited throughout the slides		
	You cover the limitations and future areas of the implementation briefly, with some interesting points around the use of this method, which gave some good insight to your excellent understanding. Your evaluation again was clear, but it could be improved further by the use of references to support your approach		
4	Well done for producing this presentation; the production level is of the highest quality and you have shown expert skills in terms of utilising technology to produce this work. I really liked the way you embedded a video into the presentation to show the CPR method	70+	Excellent presentation skills
	Your implementation approach is clearly outlined and linked with research to support your choice of method		Rationale is strong
	The rationale for the implementation of methods is strong and well planned, again linked with research where appropriate		Excellent references
	The depth shown in your implementation and evaluation of the impact of the use of the chosen method is excellent; the only area for improvement would be to try to use more references		

Annotated reading list

Ajjawi, R., Tai, J., Huu Nghia, T.L., Boud, D., Johnson, L. and Patrick, C. (2020), p. 312, *shows the important links to be made between authentic assessment and practice.*

Dexter, K., Hagler, D. and Lindell, D. (2015), p. 37, *discusses the importance of designing assessments to help you develop skills in real-world practice.*

Wiewiora, A. and Kowalkiewicz, A. (2019), p. 417, *discusses the link between assessment and practice and how important it is to develop this.*

www.youtube.com/watch?v=W8ppd2XXMjs

This video talks about the gap that can exist if your assessment is not authentic, so you could struggle to apply the theory in practice.

www.youtube.com/watch?v=DlksoRNrKE8

This video looks at the definitions of authentic assessment in more detail, with some interesting examples.

www.youtube.com/watch?v=-HvxXjoXEPs

This is an interesting video which looks at why authentic assessment is important for nursing and explains its importance.

References

Ajjawi, R., Tai, J., Huu Nghia, T.L., Boud, D., Johnson, L. and Patrick, C. (2020) Aligning assessment with the needs of work-integrated learning: the challenges of authentic assessment in a complex context. *Assessment and Evaluation in Higher Education*, 45(2), 304–16. Available at: 10.1080/02602938.2019.1639613

Koretsky, M.D., McColley, C.J., Gugel, J.L. and Ekstedt, T.W. (2022) Aligning classroom assessment with engineering practice: a design-based research study of a two-stage exam with authentic assessment. *Journal of Engineering Education (Washington, D.C.)*, 111(1), 185–213. Available at: 10.1002/jee.20436

Levi, T. and Inbar-Lourie, O. (2020) Assessment literacy or language assessment literacy: learning from the teachers. *Language Assessment Quarterly*, 17(2), 168–82. Available at: 10.1080/15434303.2019.1692347

NMC (2018) *Standards of Proficiency for Registered Nurses*. London: NMC. Available at: www.nmc.org.uk/globalassets/sitedocuments/standards/2024/standards-of-proficiency-for-nurses.pdf. Accessed: 26 June 2025.

Poindexter, K., Hagler, D. and Lindell, D. (2015) Designing authentic assessment: strategies for nurse educators. *Nurse Educator*, 40(1), 36–40. Available at: 10.1097/NNE.0000000000000091

Price, M. (2012) *Assessment Literacy: The Foundation for Improving Student Learning*. Oxford: ASKe, Oxford Centre for Staff and Learning Development.

Quinlan, K.M., Sellei, G. and Fiorucci, W. (2024) Educationally authentic assessment: reframing authentic assessment in relation to students' meaningful engagement. *Teaching in Higher Education*, 30(3), 717–34. Available at: 10.1080/13562517.2024.2394042

Wiewicra, A. and Kowalkiewicz, A. (2019) The role of authentic assessment in developing authentic leadership identity and competencies. *Assessment and Evaluation in Higher Education*, 44(3), 415–30. Available at: 10.1080/02602938.2018.1516730

Written assessments

Cariona Flaherty

Chapter aims

By the end of this chapter, you should be able to:

- explain the role of written assessments in preparing you for professional qualification;
- describe the different types of written assessments, including reflection, commonly used in nurse education;
- develop effective strategies for planning and structuring a written essay as an assessment;
- demonstrate appropriate use of academic literature, including correct citation and referencing in written assessment.

Introduction

The Royal College of Nursing (RCN, 2023, p. 1) states that 'good record keeping is a vital part of effective communication in nursing and integral to promoting safety and continuity of care for patients and clients'. The NMC Code (2018, p. 13) states nurses, midwives and nursing associates must 'keep clear and accurate records relevant to your practice'. Although patient records come in many forms the key here is that record-keeping involves writing, therefore written assessments during your training will support you in developing your writing, thinking, reading and improve your ability to articulate yourself in a professional manner. Your writing is a form of communication, and anything you write within a patient record becomes a legally binding document. In the ever-changing healthcare environment, it is imperative that you have strong communication and writing skills to be able to care and advocate for your patient, and work within the wider multidisciplinary team (Mitchell and McMillan, 2018).

Howick et al. (2024) identified that one of the most significant contributors to patient safety incidents is poor communication between patients and healthcare staff. Furthermore, Tingle (2023) identified that failure to communicate effectively and keep accurate records underpins a large portion of adverse events within healthcare, and that you are only as good as the records you keep (Hassan and Ford, 2019, cited in Tingle, 2023). The written assessments you will undertake at university may be in the form of reports, essays, reflections and case studies. Although writing may form part of oral and recorded presentations, the emphasis here is the delivery of the presentation over the writing of the slides. This chapter will address the role of written assessments in preparing you for qualification and nursing. The various types of written assessment will be discussed with a view to providing insight into how you can plan and structure your writing. We will look at using the literature in support of your writing and the basic principles of referencing, with practical examples given.

Case study: Florence, first-year student nurse, part 1

Florence is a first-year nursing student. One of Florence's first assessments is to write a 1,500 word assignment linked to a case study. Florence has not written an academic essay in several years. She feels overwhelmed and unsure how to approach academic research and is finding it difficult to understand how an essay links to clinical practice and where to start with writing. She has heard the terms 'critical analysis' and 'evidence-based practice', but is struggling to understand how to apply these concepts to her writing.

Activity 2.1   Reflection

Consider Florence's case study.

1.   Who could Florence ask for support and guidance?
2.   Where could Florence access information on how to write an academic essay?

A model answer is provided at the end of this chapter.

Written assessment and nursing practice

In nursing you will need to communicate with patients, relatives and a range of healthcare professionals, via verbal and written methods. Written communication could be in the form of patient referrals, record-keeping, or patient assessments; effective communication is imperative to ensure the safe delivery of patient care. While undertaking your nurse training, you will undertake a range of written assessments, where your lecturers will not only be assessing your level of knowledge, but also your ability to write clear and accurate records. Many students fail to recognise the connection between written assessments and clinical practice, seeing them only as a requirement to pass the course. However, in addition to written communication being essential for patient care, you will also need strong writing skills for job applications, CVs and maintaining your NMC registration. NMC revalidation, which is required every three years, involves submitting a written narrative demonstrating your ability to meet continued professional development (CPD) requirements. The next activity asks you to consider the various types of written communication you undertake in practice and the possible implications of inaccurate record-keeping.

Activity 2.2 Critical thinking

Considering your experience in practice, reflect on the following questions.

1. List all the forms of written communication you have undertaken in practice.
2. Consider the impact of how care could be compromised if your written records were not accurate, or understandable.

A model answer is provided at the end of this chapter.

Written assessments in nurse education

Having considered the links between written assessments and nursing practice, we will now consider the various type of written assessments you may be asked to undertake during your training. They may take many formats – such as, essays, dissertations, QIs, case studies, oral presentations and exams. Oral presentations will be addressed in Chapter 3, QIs in Chapter 4, dissertations in Chapter 5 and exams in Chapter 8. Therefore, this chapter will focus on essays, case studies and reflective writing.

Essays and case studies

Written essays and case studies are used widely within nurse education, where students are tasked with writing an essay about a topic or writing an essay where a patient case study is the focus. The two are similar in structure, but different in terms of focus; an essay may have a broader topic of discussion, whereas a case study may ask you to focus on a specific patient. For this book, a case study will be referred to as within a written essay – not the writing up of a case study as you would normally see in research writing. Whether it is an essay or case study, the first thing for you as a student to do, is to understand the marking criteria or assessment brief. The marking criteria will help you to understand the specifics of what your lecturer is assessing you against; for example, if the marking criteria is asking you to 'critically analyse the underlying pathophysiology with links to the case study' then you are expected to critically analyse pathophysiology and link this to the patient in the case study. Another example: if the marking criteria asks you to 'utilise supporting literature', this means your essay must be generated from your reading of the literature. For further information on understanding the marking criteria, refer to Chapter 1.

After you have reviewed the marking criteria, the next stage is to understand what the essay or case study is asking you to do. What question is being asked – for example, is it to discuss, debate, critically analyse or explain (see Table 2.1)? The verb that is used will ultimately tie to the academic year you are in, and links to Bloom's taxonomy (see Figure 2.1). Bloom's taxonomy outline the verbs used within academic assessments that increase in complexity as you move through academic years. For example, *remembering and understanding* would normally be associated with first year; *applying and analysing* would then be linked with second year; and *evaluating and creating* aligned with third year. The verbs used within assessments are not restricted to these examples, but they do offer insight into the increasing complexity of verbs used within academic assessments and associated levels of study.

Table 2.1 Keys verbs and meaning (adapted from Boyd, 2014)

Verb	Description
Analyse	Consider or critique a topic in detail
Compare	Differences and similarities
Contrast	Outline the differences only
Critique	Act of being critical
Describe	Giving the details about a topic
Discuss	Present arguments that may be for or against
Evaluate	Give the positives or negatives about a topic
Explain	Outline the reasons
Justify	Give a valid argument
Summarise	Present the main findings

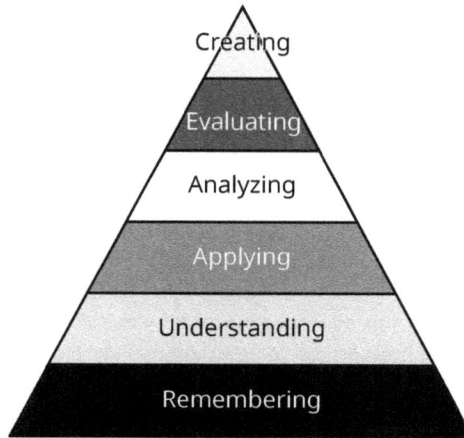

Figure 2.1 Bloom's taxonomy (My Learning Network, 2024)

Case study: Florence first-year student nurse, part 2

After Florence spoke with her lecturers she had a better understanding of how academic writing links to practice and the support that was available within her university. Florence gained new perspectives on how to approach her writing tasks and received valuable advice on improving her writing style. Despite these positive steps, Florence still feels uncertain about how to plan and structure her academic work effectively. She realises that developing these skills will take time and practice, but she is determined to make the most of the support available to her.

Activity 2.3   Critical thinking

Consider Florence's case study.

1.   What does a basic essay structure look like?
2.   How would Florence prepare to undertake a written assessment?

There is no model answer, as the answers are provided in the next section of this chapter.

Structure

Moving on from marking criteria and verbs, the next stage is to outline a proposed structure for writing an academic essay/case study. This section will present an approach to students; however, if your lecturer provides you with a clear structure, it is advised that you follow this. At a basic level every essay should have an introduction, main body and conclusion. An introduction should provide a summary of what the essay intends to discuss. This is the same for a case study, with the difference being that your introduction will refer to the study being used, providing details and then linking to the appendix, where the case study is presented in full. The key when writing an introduction is to ensure you outline all the essay requirements. For example:

> This essay will critically analyse the role of paracetamol in the management of low-grade pyrexia in pneumonia. There will be a detailed discussion on the pathophysiology of pneumonia, and its links to low-grade pyrexia. The pharmacodynamic and pharmacokinetics of paracetamol will be addressed, with reference to the literature and the role of the nurse in medicines management. This essay will conclude with a summary of the discussion and a reflection on key learning.

The above example is much shorter than is normal for essays, but your lecturers will provide details of suggested word counts; these will vary depending on overall word count. The example is only a very basic introduction to give you an idea; your introduction will be more comprehensive and based on the assessment brief you are given by your lecturers. The main body of your essay will then provide a detailed account of your knowledge and understanding of the assessment topic or case study. When writing the main body, this is where you will use the literature to support your writing; as a rule, you would:

- make an argument/statement;
- use evidence to inform your thinking;
- discuss/critique.

The important feature of the main body is your ability to use the literature to create and support your discussion. If you do not use the literature, then your essay will not meet the academic requirements of using evidence to support learning. In addition, the use of evidence underpins nursing practice – therefore, the lecturer is not only assessing your writing skills, but also your ability to use evidence to inform your practice. Once you have the main body complete, you then move on to the conclusion. The conclusion is a summary of your essay and is often described as the introduction being written as a conclusion. However, as you move into higher academic levels your conclusion will include a more in-depth summary of your learning and thoughts.

The conclusion should not contain new information, for the most part should not contain any references and normally has a similar word count to the introduction.

The above provides a basic essay/case study structure, but the writing of an essay does not solely depend on the structure; you must also plan an essay. The acronym PROCESS has been used widely to support students and writers (Lloyd, 2007). PROCESS, in this context, is *planning, referencing, organisation, composition, engineering, spelling* and *structure*.

- *Planning*

  This is the initial phase where you define the purpose of your writing, understand your audience and determine the scope of the task. You brainstorm ideas, gather research materials and create an outline to guide your writing. You attend tutorial support, schedule to see the library and academic writing support provided by your university.

  Your lecturers will provide you with a reading list for each module, a large part of writing begins with reading around the topic via books, journals, policies, etc. Your reading will then help inform your references.

- *Referencing*

  Proper referencing is essential, especially in academic writing. Here, you ensure that all sources of information are cited correctly, using the appropriate citation style (e.g. Harvard) to avoid plagiarism and give credit to original authors. Your lecturer will let you know the referencing style used within your university.

- *Organisation*

  Organising your content is crucial for clarity and flow. Arrange ideas logically, starting with an introduction, developing the main body with key arguments or points and concluding with a summary. A clear structure helps guide the reader through your work.

- *Composition*

  This is the actual drafting phase where you begin writing. Focus on expanding your outline into full sentences and paragraphs, ensuring that ideas are expressed clearly and concisely. Don't worry too much about perfection during this stage. Seek clarity from your lecturer about reading drafts and seek support from your university's academic writing team.

- *Engineering*

  This term refers to refining and reshaping your draft. This involves revising the content, improving sentence structure and ensuring your argument or narrative is well developed. You may restructure paragraphs or reword sentences for clarity.

- *Spelling*

  Careful attention to spelling, grammar, punctuation and sentence structure is crucial. Proofreading helps to ensure your work is polished and free from errors that could detract from the quality of your writing.

- *Structure*

  The final structure is about ensuring the overall organisation of your document is clear and effective. Make sure the introduction, body and conclusion work together cohesively. Verify that each section serves its intended purpose and the overall piece is well balanced.

PROCESS is just one acronym, there are several others which you will learn about at university; the key is to find one that suits your style. Having provided an overview of structuring and writing an essay, the next section will look at writing a reflective essay. While reflective writing has similarities to essay writing, there are differences – primarily that you will be asked to use a reflective model to support your writing.

Reflective assessments

Like written assessments, reflective writing links to clinical practice. Of course, it allows your writing and communication skills to be assessed, but reflection is more that than this. 'Reflection is a method of using experiential knowledge to enable professional and personal development while reinforcing continuous learning' (Gustafsson and Fagerberg, 2014, cited in Nicol and Dosser, 2016, p. 34). Reflection involves exploring who you are, examining your own values, thoughts and experience and how they all interplay. In terms of reflective writing Esterhuizen (2023) highlights that writing about your experiences helps you to learn, and create new meaning that contributes to life-long learning. Reflective writing can be difficult to begin with; it asks you to consider your experiences and explore them in your writing, while acknowledging learning and developing new ways of thinking and working. In addition to this, the literature has identified that there are three periods of reflection:

- *reflection before action*: this is thinking about what it is you want to achieve – for example, exploring the potential experience you may get while on clinical placement;
- *refection in action*: known as 'thinking on your feet', this type of reflection is normally undertaken while doing the task;
- *reflection after action*: this is reflection after the event, a retrospective view; written reflective assessments are normally this type.

(Nicol and Dosser, 2016)

Nicol and Dosser (2016) highlighted that having a range of reflective models will support your thinking and broader application of knowledge to situations. To help you begin thinking about your reflective writing assessment, this chapter will discuss two reflective models: Borton's model (1970) and Gibbs' reflective cycle (1988), which you can use to support your writing. There are several other reflective models used across nursing; your lecturer will guide you on the model they recommend. They will ask you to use one when writing your reflective module, and the principles of the PROCESS framework which was discussed previously can also continue to be used to support your reflective written assessments.

Borton's model (1970)

Borton's model was established in 1970, later adapted by Driscoll, in 2007, and then Rolfe et al. in 2010 (cited in Nicol and Dosser, 2016). Borton's model has three stages and can be used for reflection before, in and after action as follows:

- Stage 1: What?
- Stage 2: So what?
- Stage 3: Now what?

This model of reflection is a simple, structured approach to reflection that helps students consider their experiences, make sense of them and identify actions for the future. Now let's take a closer look at each stage.

Stage 1: What?

The first stage is where you would describe the situation/experience; the key is to recall the experience in an objective way. The questions you could consider asking yourself at this stage are:

- what events took place during the situation?
- who were the key people involved, what were their roles, what was your role?
- how did you feel about the outcome?
- what was your role in the situation, how did this make you feel?
- what did you observe or notice during the experience and how did this make you feel?

Stage 2: So what?

The second stage is where you analyse and explore the experience and understand why it was significant. The focus is on understanding what happened and how it affected you and others that were involved, and this is normally both on a personal and professional level. This stage will include linking with the underpinning literature; for example, if the situation were related to professional values, you would likely refer to the NMC. Your lecturer will expect you to utilise the literature at this stage to show your understanding in the context of evidence-based practice and to demonstrate your ability to think critically. The questions you could consider here are:

- what were the underlying causes?
- why did it happen in the way it did?
- how did it make you feel, during and after the event?
- what aspect of the experience went well and which areas could you improve on?
- what have you learned from this experience?
- what literature does this experience reflect or relate to?

Stage 3: Now what?

The final stage is where you identify what you will do differently based on your reflection. It focuses on specific action and planning for improvement. The questions you could consider at this stage are:

- what would you do differently if in a similar situation?
- how will you apply the learning?
- what additional training would I need to support my development?
- based on this reflection, what improvements can I make?

Bolton's reflective model is easy to follow, encourages deep thinking and can help you make sense of experiences to learn and grow. The next model of reflection is Gibbs' reflective cycle (1988, cited in Nicol and Dosser, 2016).

Gibbs' reflective cycle

Gibbs' model of reflection contains six stages: *description, feelings, evaluation, analysis, conclusion, action plan*. Gibbs' approach allows for a deeper analysis of the experience, identifying an action plan for future personal and professional development. Now let's look at each stage of Gibbs' reflective cycle.

Description

The first stage involves describing the experience, providing factual and detailed account to set the context for reflection. You could consider the following questions:

- what happened?
- where and when?
- who was involved?
- what did you and others do?

Feelings

The second stage is where you would explore your thoughts and emotions about the experience. The purpose of this stage is to help you to acknowledge and understand your emotional response and how your feelings may have influenced your actions during the situation. The questions you may ask yourself are:

- what were you feeling before, during and after the situation?
- how did you feel?
- how did others feel/show emotion?
- how did your feelings impact the situation?

Evaluation

The third stage involves evaluating your experience by looking at both positive and negative aspects. This is where you start to assess what worked well and what didn't. Questions to ask:

- what was good about the experience?
- what didn't go well and why?
- what aspects were effective or ineffective?
- how did others contribute positively or negatively to the experience?

Analysis

The fourth stage is where you work on analysing the situation to understand why things happened the way they did. You try to reflect on the reasons behind the positive and negative aspects and start to make sense of the experience. Questions for you to consider:

- why did things happen the way they did?
- what factors influenced the outcome (e.g. skills, knowledge, environment)?
- how did your actions or the actions of others affect the result?
- what could have been done differently?

Conclusion

The fifth stage involves arriving at conclusions about what you've learned. This stage is where you would determine what you have learned from the experience and how you will improve future practice. Questions to consider at this stage are:

- what have you learned from this experience?
- what skills or knowledge do you need to develop?
- how could this situation be avoided or improved in the future?

Action plan

The final stage is focused on creating an action plan for future situations. This is about taking what you've learned and deciding how you'll approach similar situations differently to improve outcomes. The questions you could consider are:

- what will you do differently next time?
- how will you apply the lessons learned?
- what actions will you take to develop the skills or knowledge needed?

Irrespective of what reflective model you chose, when asked to write a reflective essay you will be required to follow a model. Look at the next activity and begin to think about how you would use a reflective model.

Activity 2.4   Reflection

1. Select one of the above reflective models and evaluate an experience you had in practice.
2. Why did you choose that specific reflective model for this activity?

As this is a personal reflection, no model answer is provided at the end of this chapter.

Basic principles of referencing and plagiarism

For all assessments you will be asked to utilise the underpinning literature to support your work, therefore you must learn to write citations and reference correctly. Citations appear in the body of the essay to show where specific information came from such as direct quotations. References appear at the end of your work in a separate section titled *references* or *reference list*.

Flaherty and Taylor (2024) identified that referencing helps students to make academic arguments, provide evidence of quality in written assessments and demonstrates professionalism. Each university will be aligned with a specific reference style, such as Harvard or American Psychological Association (APA). To support you with referencing Cite Them Right (2024) offers guidance online and in book format (see Annotated reading list). Remember – all resources that you use, such as books, websites, journals and videos must be referenced.

It is important that you reference all sources of evidence you use; doing this will ensure you avoid plagiarism. Price (2014, p. 46) identifies plagiarism as 'the representation of others' words in a piece of coursework or academic assignment as one's own, without clear reference to the source and/or failure to represent the words of others as a quotation'. With the increase in the use of artificial intelligence (AI), it is worth noting here that using AI to write your assignment is also seen as plagiarism. Your university will have specific guidelines on what is and is not plagiarism, breach of which would be regarded as academic misconduct. First-year students often unintentionally plagiarise – often due to academic naivety, being new to university. However, whether intentional or unintentional, plagiarism will result in academic penalties; such penalties could result in the failing of an assessment all the way through to expulsion from the university. Plagiarism is linked to honesty and a student's academic integrity. For a nursing student, academic integrity also aligns with the NMC Code (2018); ensuring you reference correctly and in line with your university reference systems will ensure you uphold this code. Price (2014) discusses several ways you can avoid plagiarism as follows:

- save your literature searches and keep accurate notes;
- learn how to paraphrase – put what you read into your own words;
- use quotation marks correctly;
- seek support from your lecturer and academic writing support services at your university.

Activity 2.5   Evidence-based writing

Using the Harvard referencing style, answer the following questions (use Cite Them Write, 2024, to help you):

1.   How do you reference a journal?
2.   How do you reference a printed book?

A model answer is provided at the end of this chapter.

Having a clear understanding of how to reference any source you use within your assessment will ensure you avoid plagiarism and subsequent academic misconduct issues.

Conclusion

Written assessments play a crucial role in preparing nursing students for qualification by developing critical thinking, clinical reasoning and communication skills essential for professional practice. By familiarising yourself with the different types of written assessments – such as essays, case studies and reflective writing – you can effectively demonstrate knowledge and understanding of key nursing concepts. Proper planning and structuring of these assessments are vital for success, as is the ability to apply referencing principles and avoid plagiarism – fundamental to maintaining academic integrity. This chapter began by exploring the connection between written assessments, clinical practice and effective communication. It provided an overview of assessment-related verbs and guidance on structuring an academic essay. Two widely used reflective models were examined, highlighting how they can be applied to written reflective assessments. The chapter concluded with a brief discussion on referencing and the importance of avoiding plagiarism.

Brief outline answers

Activity 2.1 Reflection

1. Who could Florence ask for support and guidance?

Florence could speak with her lecturers, peers, librarian and academic writing support team at her university.

2. Where could Florence access information on how to write an academic essay?

Writing guidance will be provided by Florence's lecturers, and the library services will have several support structures in place to support students, such as 1:1 support and academic writing workshops.

Activity 2.2 Critical thinking

1. List all the forms of written communication you have undertaken in practice.

Reports, audits, observation recording, referrals, patient records/notes, assessments, intake and output charts, drugs charts.

2. Consider the impact of how care could be compromised if your written records were not accurate, or understandable.

Inaccurate records could compromise patient care and lead to incorrect actions or care being missed. Your writing also needs to be legible so that others can clearly understand what you have written.

Activity 2.5 Evidence-based writing

1. How do you reference a journal?

    -   Author (surname followed by initials)
    -   Year of publication (in round brackets)
    -   Title of article (in single quotation marks)
    -   Total of journal (in italics – capitalise the first letter of each significant word)
    -   Issue: volume
    -   Page reference

2. How do you reference a printed book?

    -   Author
    -   Year of publication (in round brackets)
    -   Title (in italics)
    -   Edition
    -   Place of publication: Publisher
    -   Series and volume number (if available)

Cite Them Right (2024)

Annotated further reading

Biggam, J. (2020) *Succeeding with Your University Essay: A Step-by-step Handbook.* London: McGraw Hill.

A complete step-by-step guide that delves deeper into academic writing at university level.

Price, B. (2017) Improving nurses' level of reflection. *Nursing Standard*, 32(1), 52–63.

This article provides a good overview of reflective practice for nurses.

References

Boyd, C. (2014) *Study Skills for Nurses*. Oxford: Wiley Blackwell.

Cite Them Right (2024) Available at: www.citethemrightonline.com/

Esterhuizen, P. (2023) *Reflective Practice in Nursing*. London: Learning Matters.

Flaherty, C. and Taylor, M. (2024) *Developing Academic Writing Skills for Nursing Associates.* 2nd Edition. London: Learning Matters.

Howick, J., Bennett-Weston, A., Solomon, J., Nockels, K., Bostock, J. and Keshtkar, L. (2024) How does communication affect patient safety? Protocol for a systematic review and logic model. *British Medical Journal*, 14, e085312. Available at: 10.1136/bmjopen-2024-085312

Lloyd, M. (2007) Developing academic writing skills: the PROCESS framework. *Nursing Standard*, 21(40), 50–6.

Mitchell, K. and McMillan, D. (2018) A curriculum-wide assessment of writing self-efficacy in a baccalaureate nursing program. *Nurse Education Today*, 70, 20–7.

My Learning Network (2024) *Bloom's Taxonomy*. Available at: https://mylearningnetwork.com/ blooming-as-a-learner/. Accessed: 3 September 2024.

Nicol, J.S. and Dosser, I. (2016) Understanding reflective practice. *Nursing Standard*, 30(36), 34–42.

NMC (2018) *The Code: Professional Standards of Practice and Behaviour for Nurses, Midwives and Nursing Associates*. London: NMC.

Price, B. (2014) Avoiding plagiarism: guidance for nursing students. *Nursing Standard*, 28(26), 45–51.

Royal College of Nursing (RCN) (2023) *Record Keeping: The Facts*. Available at: www.rcn.org.uk/ Professional-Development/publications/rcn-record-keeping-uk-pub-011-016. Accessed: 26 June 2025.

Tingle, J. (2023) Facing the consequences of poor record keeping and communication. *British Journal of Nursing*, 32, 3. Available at: www.britishjournalofnursing.com/content/patient-safety/facing-the-consequences-of-poor-record-keeping-and-communication. Accessed 12 September 2024.

Presentations

Cariona Flaherty

Chapter aims

By the end of this chapter, you should be able to:

- discuss the various approaches to presentations;
- link presentations as a means of assessment to nursing practice;
- identify how to plan and deliver a narrated presentation;
- discuss how to undertake and deliver an individual or group presentation;
- highlight the benefits and challenges with delivering a group presentation and strategies to support you in overcoming these.

Introduction

As we learned in Chapter 1, there's been a move towards authentic assessments that mirror real-life nursing practice. This means that you'll encounter a wide variety of different assessments during your nursing training, including essays, exams, narrated and/or group presentations; it's presentations that we now turn to in Chapter 3. Assessments are designed to measure your understanding and application of taught content to patient care, while also providing an opportunity for you to display your learning. In nurse education, presentations have become a fundamental method of assessment, offering an authentic approach to demonstrate knowledge and skill. Presentations can be narrated or oral; they might be completed individually or as a group. Moutrey (2020, p. 71) identified that 'from student life, having to produce a presentation, either individually or as a group, through to the need, once qualified, to be able to present information to others in a team or to management reporting on a study, audit or practice' is imperative.

Undertaking a presentation is a means of communication and, in line with the NMC (2024), 'effective communication is central to the provision of safe and compassionate person-centred care'. Upon qualifying as a nurse, you must be able to demonstrate a diverse range of communication skills and adapt your communication style to support people that may have special communication needs. Chiang et al. (2022) highlighted that good presentation skills, although imperative for quality patient–nurse communication, also are advantageous for promotion, leadership and professional development. It is for these reasons that you're assessed via presentations.

This chapter will explore various types of presentation with a focus on narrated, individual and group, highlighting their relevance to nursing practice. We will discuss the planning and delivery of presentations, as well as approaches you can consider to effectively approach both individual and group presentations – finalising with an overview of the benefits and challenges associated with group presentations and strategies to overcome any issues. Before we begin, let's look at a student case study and questions that may arise if you are a first-year student nurse about to undertake a presentation as part of an assessment.

Case study: Gloria, first-year student nurse

Gloria is a first-year student nurse. One of her module assessments is a 15-minute narrated presentation. The topic is *scientific principles*, and the focus is on a case study from clinical practice. This is the first time Gloria has undertaken a narrated presentation as part of her nursing studies and, understandably, Gloria is quite nervous. In preparation for undertaking this type of assessment Gloria has sought support from various sources. Her lecturer has advised her on the requirements of the presentation, providing clear guidelines and expectations. The librarian has provided access to numerous resources, including books, journals and online databases. Additionally, the IT department has supported Gloria with a step-by-step guide on how to access and use the various recording software available. This comprehensive support has helped to relieve some of her worries about presenting, allowing her to focus on delivering a well-prepared and confident presentation.

Activity 3.1   Reflection

Consider Gloria's case study.

1. Why are presentation skills important in nursing?
2. Why do you think Gloria is worried about undertaking this assessment?

A model answer is provided at the end of this chapter.

Presentation skills in nursing

Hadfield-Law (2001, p. 1208) defined an effective presentation as the 'ability to communicate a message to an audience in a way that results in a change in understanding or opinion'. Delivering presentations will confidently help you to enhance your communication skills – this is important as clear communication is crucial for safe patient care and supports nurses' professional development, which Vollman (2005, p. 67) describes as the 'best collateral for future career success'. Nevertheless, presenting can evoke anxiety among students, primarily due to fear of public speaking.

Grieve et al. (2021) highlighted that fear of public speaking, coupled with social anxiety disorder, can significantly increase a student's worry – more so than when undertaking written assessments or group work. There is often a variety of reasons why you might worry about undertaking presentations, such as: lack of confidence in public speaking, not fully understanding the requirements of the assessment and pressure to pass the assessment. Your lecturers will have developed a range of strategies to support you in undertaking presentations, either individually or as a group, narrated or oral. The next section will discuss the difference between a narrated presentation and a live presentation, highlighting a step-by-step approach for success in both.

Activity 3.2   Reflection

Imagine that you have been asked to deliver a 15-minute narrated presentation and you are unsure how to begin this assessment task. The following video provides introductory tips for undertaking nursing presentations. Watch the video and reflect on how you could use this information to support your success with undertaking this assessment task.

1.   Forde-Johnson (2023) *Nursing Presentation for a University Assessment: 7 Tips to Improve Your Marks!* Available at: https://youtu.be/P9PQrBLIpqs.

As this is a personal reflection, no model answer is provided at the end of this chapter.

Narrated presentations vs live presentations

The increased presence of online teaching since the COVID-19 pandemic has resulted in the introduction of narrated presentations as an assessment approach within nurse education. In comparison to the traditional mode of 'live' presenting, which is oral and in person, narrated presentations are online and provide a recorded narration of your presentation. A narrated presentation primarily assesses your understanding of taught content and ability to apply it to patient care, but your communication skills and, more importantly, your digital literacy skills are also assessed. Health Education England (HEE) and the Royal College of Nursing (RCN) (2017, p. 3) highlight that 'it's no longer possible to think about digital literacy as either purely technical proficiency or just something "other people" do'. Everyone working with healthcare requires the sound digital competence and 'people who have better digital literacy tend to have more positive attitudes and behaviours to adopting new technologies' (HEE and RCN, 2017, p. 5). Therefore, undertaking a narrated presentation as part of an assessment will support you in developing the necessary skill set to utilise technology in support of learning and professional practice.

Foulkes (2015) and Kapterev (2012, cited in Foulkes) have described some guiding principles that are useful to keep in mind when preparing for your own presentations (see Tables 3.1 and 3.2), but it's worth noting that they don't put much emphasis on the use of narrated presentations. This section will combine the work of Kapterev and Foulkes by applying their principles to undertaking a narrated presentation.

Table 3.1   Five principles to structure presentations (Foulkes, 2015)

	Description
Principle 1	Define what you are trying to achieve with your presentation
Principle 2	Define your audience and what it needs to know
Principle 3	Access how technology can add value to your presentation
Principle 4	Work out how principles 1–3 affect the structure and timing of your presentation
Principle 5	Define how you want to come across while you are presenting

Table 3.2   Seven principles for presentations (Kapterev, 2012, cited in Foulkes, 2015)

	Description
Principle 1	*What* is far more important than *how* (content)
Principle 2	Peer-to-peer communication (sharing rather than persuading)
Principle 3	Please interrupt me (presentations are conversations)
Principle 4	Let's make the small print big (do not attempt to hide problems)
Principle 5	You are the hero (be transparent and honest)
Principle 6	My target audience is simply *humans* (create an emotional connection)
Principle 7	Technology matters (learn how to use devices to your advantage)

Step-by-step guide to undertaking a narrated or live presentation

The following steps apply to both live and narrated presentations. Any differences between the two formats will be noted within each step.

Step 1 Understand the assessment details

The first step when undertaking any presentation is to understand what is being asked of you, or what the purpose of your presentation is (Hadfield-Law, 2001). Your lecturer will provide assessment criteria and details and will provide a number of opportunities for you to clarify and re-clarify that you should take advantage of if you have any uncertainty. A good starting point is to review how marks are being awarded and use this to support the structure of your presentation.

Step 2 Research the topic

With any assessment you undertake, understanding the topic is key. This step involves reading around the topic, looking at the literature and using the literature well within the presentation to support the narration. Use of and application of the underpinning literature is required across all assessment tasks within higher education over all years of your programme.

It is also key at this stage to know your audience and the academic level required. For example, in your first year, when you'll be at level 4, assessments are used in the context of *describing*. In contrast, by your third year, at level 6, you'll need to provide a greater depth of critical analysis.

The following provides an approach to researching the topic:

1   review existing knowledge from lectures and your own notes;
2   review the web – for example, Google Scholar™;
3   complete a review of the literature (refer to Chapter 5) – including articles, books, policies and videos;
4   create a mind-map to organise the above and identify what is relevant to the aim of your presentation and what is not;
5   start preparing the content of your slide and allow enough time to edit content several times;
6   rehearse your presentation out loud as much as possible, ensuring you are familiar with the content.

(Chivers and Shoolbred, 2007; Levin and Topping, 2008; Foulkes, 2015)

Step 3 Know your audience

Whether you are presenting to one person, a group of people, or narrating your representation you must know your audience. Levin and Topping (2008) suggest that you ask yourself the following two questions:

1. *Who is the audience?*

    For you, as student, your audience will include your lecturers and may include a service user or a peer. You will pitch your presentation to meet the learning outcomes of the assessment, and your lecturers, peers and service users will all have varying degrees of background knowledge.

2. *Why does your audience need to hear this presentation?*

    While studying the overarching purpose of your presentation will form part of the assessment process.

Understanding the above will support you with preparing and planning your presentation, as well as the level of knowledge required.

Step 4 Prepare and structure the presentation

Use the following tips when using PowerPoint to design your presentation to make sure your slides are readable:

*   use a readable font – plain and simple, and the same font throughout;
*   recommended font size 24 for main headings, 22 for subheadings and 20/18 for the text thereafter. Whichever you choose, you should remain consistent throughout;
*   do not overuse colour – less is more; some of your audience may be colour blind;
*   use visual aids to enhance your presentation – images when used wisely can be engaging;
*   use bullet points where possible.

These are relatively basic points to remember. Table 3.3 outlines a more comprehensive summary of guidance on designing your presentation.

Table 3.3 Tips for preparing your PowerPoint (adapted from, Foulkes, 2015, p. 55; Vollman, 2005, p. 71)

	Description
1	PowerPoint will not provide a structure; you need to be clear on your content and structure before using PowerPoint
2	With templates, ensure the design does not interfere with seeing the text
3	Avoid reading directly from the slides
4	Use pictures and graphics wisely – graphics on the left side of slide
5	Keep slides plain and avoid overuse of background design – use consistent colour throughout
6	One concept and one theme per slide
7	Keep text to a minimum and use your own knowledge to support the content – general rule, five words in the title, seven words per line and seven lines per slide

Once you have finalised the design, the next stage is to establish a clear structure, similar to writing an academic essay. Every presentation should start with a clear introduction that introduces you as the presenter, outlines the topic and provides an overview of the presentation. Following the introduction, you present the main content (the body of the presentation) and then conclude with a summary of key points. This summary is crucial as it allows you to recap the content succinctly. Your final slide should list the references used throughout the presentation, which is especially important when the presentation is used as part of an assessment. If you are presenting live, allocate time for questions at the end. This step is not necessary for a narrated presentation submission.

Step 5 Accessing and using recording technology (narrated presentations)

When undertaking a narrated presentation, understanding how to use technology is fundamental. A narrated presentation can be recorded using the functionality within PowerPoint, or more commonly using Zoom™, or Teams™. Your university may have alternative modes of technology to support the narration of presentations, but, for this book, the use of PowerPoint and Zoom will be the focus.

- *PowerPoint*

Let's begin with a step-by-step run through recording using PowerPoint:

1. within your PowerPoint presentation, using the top toolbar click on *slideshow*;
2. from the slideshow drop down menu, click record *from beginning*;
3. make sure your microphone settings are on (top right-hand corner settings);
4. to begin recording select *record* (top left-hand corner settings);
5. begin speaking after the countdown;
6. you can use the arrows on the left- and right-hand side of the presentation to move the slides;
7. once you have completed your recording, click *replay* to hear your narrated presentation.

The following YouTube™ video provides a narrated video recording of the above steps: *How to Record Presentations in Microsoft PowerPoint* (Microsoft, 2021). Available at: https://youtu.be/bP9VJo3s8Gw

- *Zoom*

Recording a narrated presentation can be easily achieved using the screen-share and record function on Zoom as follows:

1. log into your Zoom account and set up a new online meeting;
2. open the meeting, ensuring your microphone and camera are *unmuted*;
3. open your presentation in the background and share screen;
4. press the *record* function on the top of the Zoom task bar;
5. you can save your recording to your computer; ensure you can locate the file accordingly.

The following YouTube video provides a narrated video recording of the above steps: Stratvert, K. (2020) *How to Screen Record on Zoom*. Available at: https://youtu.be/yii4M52o4SE?si=eLrb yvgrrluK2atU

Using the functionality of recording your narration on either PowerPoint or Zoom will depend on the compatibility with your university's online learning platform; your lecturer will discuss this with you and provide guidance. Remember that once you have recorded your narration you will need to upload it to the university's online learning platform for submission. This is an incredibly important step; again your lecturer will provide guidance on this for you.

Step 6 Practising, timing and presenting your presentation

Although preparing the content for your presentation is crucial, the manner in which you deliver and present it is just as significant (Foulkes, 2015). One of the first steps here is considering your own voice. Pitch your tone at the right level, speak slowly and clearly and try not to rush. Smile and develop a rapport with your audience; use the room to move around if you need to. For narrated presentations, recording your presentations several times will help you find a slow, clear voice which will also support you when presenting live. Watch how your lecturers present and if opportunities arise to sit in on conference or other presentations please do take advantage of this.

Once you have found your voice and tone, you need to time your presentation and rehearse several times. Timing your presentation is crucial as your summative assessments will have a time limit which you must adhere to. Here are some 'top tips' to support you in delivering your assessment:

- prepare and practise over and over;
- consider the tone, pitch and speed of your voice throughout;
- take it slow and remember to breathe;
- use appropriate body language and eye contact to engage with your audience;
- smile when appropriate;
- finish with a positive note and allow time for questions;
- be confident in yourself!

(Adapted from Van Emden and Becker, 2016)

Activity 3.3   Reflection

Using the above information for *Step 6 Practising, timing and presenting your presentation*, consider the following questions.

1.   Reflect on a presentation you attended where you were disinterested: what were the reasons for this?
2.   Reflect on a presentation that you found interesting and engaging: what were the reasons for this?

As this is a personal reflection, no model answer is provided at the end of this chapter.

Now that we've reviewed the main steps involved in preparing presentations, the next section will outline the typical criteria used to evaluate these presentations.

What is being assessed in presentations?

Presentations as a means of assessment differ significantly from, for example, writing an essay – often causing a degree of uncertainty for students. However, there will be clear criteria used to assess and grade your presentation. The most commonly assessed aspects of a student's presentation are:

1.   the content is accurate, factual and up to date;
2.   the structure is consistent, with a clear introduction, main body and summary;
3.   effective use of visual aids to support your presentation;
4.   vocal delivery and audience engagement;
5.   utilising prepared notes;
6.   time keeping;
7.   integration of the literature within the presentation and providing an accurate reference list;
8.   ability to answer questions effectively.

Activity 3.4   Critical thinking

Review the assessment (marking) criteria you have been given for your own presentation and make a list of what is being asked.

1.   How does this compare with the above section?

As this is an individualised activity, no model answer is provided at the end of this chapter.

You may be asked to undertake your presentation individually or as a group with your peers. With this come benefits and challenges, which we now look at in more detail.

Group presentations

The guidance provided in the previous sections on completing and preparing for individual and narrated presentations applies to group presentations too; however, additional considerations must be addressed when presenting as a group. Like individual presentations, group presentations will look to assess your communication skills, but, more importantly, your ability to work within a team – teams that work together well and communicate effectively perform better and provide better patient care (Creighton and Smart, 2022). Additionally, the NMC (2024) outlines that to practise effectively nurses must work with and support their colleagues.

There are several advantages to undertaking a presentation as part of a group:

- workload is shared;
- range of individual abilities and sharing;
- ability to demonstrate your ability to perform within a group;
- working within a group is a transferrable skill;
- increased group performance;
- social opportunities;
- reflects practice working.

However, there are also several challenges to working within a group:

- different opinions and talents;
- lack of clear goals;
- role uncertainty;
- conflict within the team;
- varying levels of commitment.

(Chivers and Shoolbred, 2007; Van Emden and Becker, 2016)

Let's look at an activity around the benefits and challenges of working within a team.

Activity 3.5　Critical thinking

Think of a time you worked as part of a team and reflect on the following questions:

1. What were the benefits of working within the team?
2. What were the challenges with working within the team?
3. How did you overcome the challenges?

A model answer is provided at the end of this chapter.

Having completed this activity let's now move on to looking at the stages of group development.

Stages of group development

Understanding the stages of group development is an important aspect of learning when tasked to work within groups. Tuckman and Jensen (1977, cited in Chivers and Shoolbred, 2007), provides a five-stage approach to group development as follows:

- forming
- storming
- norming
- performing
- adjourning.

Now let's look at each stage in the context of working on a group presentation.

Forming

This is the stage where your lecturer informs you of the group you will be working with and the assessment details. Getting to know each other and sharing experience will support with identifying roles. For example, at this stage you will start by contacting your group and setting out an initial date to meet.

Storming

This is where ideas on structuring and designing the presentation start to take shape. Conflicts often arise at this stage due to possible resistance within the team due to conflicting ideas and personality type. It can be the most challenging time as stronger personalities may dominate and take the lead. For example, at this stage, the leader may be appointed by the group and you all start to brainstorm ideas, identifying clear roles and tasks within the group.

Norming

During the norming stage, the team begins to establish norms, cohesion and a sense of belonging. There is increased cooperation, roles are set, communication improves and conflicts are resolved. If, at this stage, you find that conflict remains within the team, it would be advisable to seek guidance from your lecturer. You should all be clear about your roles – such as to design the presentation layout and identify images to use.

Performing

This fourth stage sees the team moving beyond any conflict and establishing effective working relationships. Members are flexible and the team moves towards producing the content for the presentation. Roles are clearly defined and there is a sense of confidence within the team. This stage would also include the delivery of the presentation and completion of the assessment task. For example, as a group you would be ready to deliver the presentation, each knowing what aspects they are responsible for.

Adjourning

The final stage is normally where the team would have a debrief. As part of the presentation, you may be asked to reflect on your experience of working as part of a team and how you will use this experience to support you in practice. Reflection on what could have been done differently and what might work better for future projects is also an important aspect of this stage. You may be asked by your lecturers to write a 100-word reflection on working as part of a group, or this may be one of the questions you are asked to consider at the end of your presentation (Chivers and Shoolbred, 2007).

Conflict, in one form or another, can be one of the more challenging parts of working in a group. However, it can also be a valuable learning experience. By facing and working through conflict, you're building the resilience and skills you need to handle similar situations more confidently in the future. Let's look at some top tips for dealing with conflict within a group.

Top tips: dealing with conflict

1. *Stay objective*: try to remember the reason why you are working in a group and focus on the issues rather than your emotions.
2. *Listen*: allow all the group to speak without interrupting; this will ensure everyone feels valued.
3. *Understand*: try and understand the cause of the conflict; for example, is the issue around poor group communication?
4. *Compromise*: suggest ways to adjust group roles and encourage the group to collectively agree any changes.
5. *Reflect and learn*: use this experience to learn for the future; as a nurse you will always have to work within a group in some ways.

But remember, if all the above fails in resolving the conflict reach out to your lecturer who may offer some helpful advice or perhaps could act as a mediator.

Hopefully, by this stage of the chapter you have a good understanding of how to undertake a presentation as part of an assessment. As mentioned previously, despite all help, tips and guidance, the anxiety you feel about presenting may remain. To help, let's look at some top tips which may help you to overcome some of this anxiety.

Top tips: dealing with presentation anxiety

1. *Prepare thoroughly*: know the content of what you are about to present inside out. This includes organising your presentation as you would an essay: introduction, main body and conclusion.
2. *Anticipate potential questions*: write out some questions you may be asked and pre-prepare answers. Seek guidance from your lecturers as they may have pre-planned generic questions that all students will be asked.
3. *Practise*: rehearse out loud, alone or with peers or family. It can help to record yourself presenting and then review the recording and note areas in your presentation that may need revising.
4. *Try to calm your nerves*: take a deep breath, allow yourself to the count of three and commit to moving on. Use positive self-talk; remember, you've got this! Some students find it helpful to visualise themselves presenting a confident and successful presentation – it can help with promoting a positive mindset.
5. *Try to focus on the end goal*: don't try to be perfect; instead focus on delivering the content of the presentation – try to think of yourself as teaching your lecturers ... they want to know more about your topic.
6. *Engage your lecturers*: make eye contact (every so often), speak slowly and clearly. If you find yourself speaking too fast, take a pause and reset. Remember to smile – this is your work and you should be very proud!
7. *Bullet points*: don't overload your slides, use bullet points and keep it simple.
8. *Reflect*: after the presentation, take some time to reflect and congratulate yourself – you've done it!

Conclusion

This chapter began by highlighting the growing use of presentations as a method of assessment in nurse education, with a focus on their relevance to clinical practice. Presentations as a mode of assessment provide you with the opportunity to enhance your communication skills and utilise evidence-based practice. This chapter explored the various types of presentations, which tend to be live or narrated. Guidance was provided on how to plan and deliver a successful narrated presentation, including structuring content, using visual images effectively and recording presentations with professionalism. This chapter also covered the process of preparing for both individual and group presentations, outlining the importance of time management, allocations of roles within the group and rehearsing. Strategies to overcome the potential challenges of group conflict included using clear communication, setting group expectations and the importance of listening. This chapter concluded by providing some top tips for overcoming presentation anxiety to support you in successfully delivering your presentation.

Brief outline answers

Activity 3.1 Reflection

1.   Why are presentation skills important in nursing?

They help you prepare for future employment, enhance your communication and team working skills and provide opportunities for you to link theory to practice.

2.   Why do you think Gloria is worried about undertaking this assessment?

Presenting to an audience can be quite daunting; often students feel anxious. Your lecturers will support you, in addition to the tips on how to overcome presentation anxiety included in this chapter.

Activity 3.5 Critical thinking

Think of a time you worked as part of a team and reflect on the following questions:

1.   What were the benefits of working within the team?

Provides an opportunity to work with and learn from others, and provides exposure to a variety of knowledge and experience.

2.   What were the challenges with working within the team?

Conflict and lots of opinions, which can make navigating the team dynamics difficult.

3.   How did you overcome the challenges?

Clear communication, actively listen, reassigning roles and valuing everyone's opinion.

Annotated further reading

Foulkes, M. (2015) Presentation skills for nurses. *Nursing Standard*, 29(5), 52–8.

This is an easy-to-follow guide outlining presentation skills for nurses.

Hatchett, R. (2024) How to give an effective conference presentation. *Nursing Standard*, 10.7748/ns.2024.e12389.

Although this article relates to conference presentations, it includes techniques on preparing presentation slides and communication strategies which you may find helpful.

References

Chiang Y.-C., Lee, H.-C., Chu, T.-L., Wu, C.-L. and Hsiao, T.-C. (2022) Development and validation for the oral presentation evaluation scale (OPES) for nursing students. *BMC Medical Education*, 22(318) 1–11.

Chivers, B. and Shoolbred, M. (2017) *A Student's Guide to Presentations: Making Your Own Presentation Count.* London: Sage.

Creighton, L. and Smart, A. (2022) Professionalism in nursing 2: working as part of a team. *Nursing Times*, 118(5), 27–30.

Forde-Johnson, C. (2023) *Nursing Presentation for a University Assessment: 7 Tips to Improve Your Marks!* Available at: https://youtu.be/P9PQrBLIpqs. Accessed: 27 June 2025.

Foulkes, M. (2015) Presentation skills for nurses. *Nursing Standard*, 29(5), 52–8.

Grieve, E., Woodley, S., Hunt, E. and McKay, A. (2021) Student fears of oral presentations and public speaking in higher education: a qualitative survey. *Journal of Further and Higher Education*, 45(9), 1281–93.

Hadfield-Law, L. (2001) Presentation skills for nurses: how to prepare more effectively. *British Journal of Nursing*, 10(18), 1208–11.

Health Education England (HEE) and Royal College of Nursing (RCN) (2017) *Improving Digital Literacy.* Available at: Improving-digital-literacy (3).pdf. Accessed 9 June 2024.

Levin, P. and Topping, G. (2008) *Perfect Presentations.* New York: Open University Press.

Microsoft (2021) *How to Record Presentations in Microsoft PowerPoint.* Available at: https://youtu.be/bP9VJ03s8Gw. Accessed 25 May 2024.

Moutrey, S. (2020) *The Healthcare Students' Academic Companion.* London: Open University Press.

NMC (2024) *Standards of Proficiencies for Registered Nurses.* Available at: standards-of-proficiency-for-nurses.pdf (nmc.org.uk). Accessed: 2 June 2024.

Stratvert, K. (2020) *How to Screen Record on Zoom.* Available at: https://youtu.be/yii4M5204SE?si=eLrbyvgrrluK2atU. Accessed on 25 May 2024.

Van Emden, J. and Becker, L. (2016) *Presentation Skills for Students.* London: Palgrave.

Vollman, K.M. (2005) Enhancing presentation skills for the advanced practice nurse. *AACN Clinical Issues*, 16(1), 67–77.

Quality improvement

Cariona Flaherty

Chapter aims

By the end of this chapter, you should be able to:

- discuss the meaning of *quality improvement* (QI);
- address the importance of QI within healthcare;
- identify the underlining principles of QI;
- outline the approaches to undertaking a QI project;
- discuss how to undertake QI as an assessment.

Introduction

The Health Foundation (2021, p. 3) highlights that QI:

> is about giving the people closest to issues affecting care quality the time, permission, skills and resources they need to solve them. It involves a systematic and coordinated approach to solving a problem using specific methods and tools with the aim of bringing about a measurable improvement.

Healthcare organisations emphasise the benefits of nurses engaging in QI activities. Participating in QI provides nurses with valuable opportunities to take a leadership role in driving change, ranging from enhancing individual patient care to transforming services across complex healthcare environments (Backhouse and Ogunlayi, 2020). As a student you will only ever be asked to consider a QI project proposal, as to undertake a full QI in practice would require ethics approval and a wider research team. However, undertaking a QI project as a means of assessment will support you to develop the necessary skills to work on QI projects post-qualification. This chapter aims to discuss the concept of QI and its significance in the context of nursing care. Conducting a QI as part of your nursing course will be explored by focusing on the principles and the approaches involved. Reference will be made to a case study throughout the chapter, and there will be several activities included to further support your learning.

What is QI?

The Institute of Medicine (1990, cited in Health Foundation, 2021, p. 6) defines quality as 'the degree to which health services for individuals and populations increase the likelihood of desired health outcomes and are consist with current professional knowledge'. This means that healthcare should provide safe, effective care that is patient-centred and underpinned by up-to-date knowledge and expertise. QI is a process by which substandard care and healthcare practice can be improved. As a student you will have up-to-date knowledge from your training and you have a responsibility to use this knowledge to improve and drive high-quality care. This is reflected by the NMC (2018, p. 26) whereby, at the point of registration, nurses must be able 'to demonstrate an understanding of the principles of improvement methodologies, participate in all stages of audit activity and identify appropriate QI strategies'.

The King's Fund (2017, p. 3) suggests that QI in healthcare is 'based on the principle of health care organisations and staff continuously trying to improve how they work and the quality of care and outcomes for patients'. QI in nursing focuses on enhancing patient outcomes, improving care processes and ensuring that nursing practices are efficient, safe and effective. In 2021, towards the end of the third wave of COVID-19, Ruth May launched the professional nurse advocate (PNA) training programme, which was recognised as 'the start of a critical point of recovery: for patients, for services and for our workforce' (NHS England, 2023). The PNA is a professional clinical leadership and advocacy role that supports staff through a 'continuous quality improvement process that builds personal and professional clinical leadership, improves the quality of care delivered and supports professional revalidation' (NHS England, 2023). The recognition at this point was that QI was fundamental to the NHS's recovery post-COVID-19. Let's look at a student case study, where a QI project proposal formed part of their third-year summative assessment.

Case study: Samuel, third-year student nurse, part 1

Samuel is in the final year of his nursing course; he has been asked to write a 5,000-word QI project proposal. The assessment guidelines have asked Samuel to consider an area of practice which he thinks requires improvement. During his clinical placements, he has noticed that the documentation of patient observations was sometimes inconsistent or even incomplete. This inconsistency could lead to miscommunication among the team and potentially impact patient outcomes. Samuel wants to look at improving the documenting of patient observations by nursing staff. He has never undertaken a QI as a means of assessment and is struggling with how to begin working on his QI proposal.

Activity 4.1   Reflection

1. Consider Samuel's case study. Where could Samuel find out information on how to undertake a QI?
2. Who could Samuel speak with?

A model answer is provided at the end of this chapter.

Examples of QI initiatives in nursing might focus on reducing infection rates, improving patient safety, enhancing patient satisfaction, or improving communication to patients and their families. Activity 4.2 will help you begin to think about your experience in placements and how you might work to improve practice.

Activity 4.2   Critical thinking

Reflecting on your clinical placements consider the following questions.

1. Did you see areas of practice which could be improved?
2. Why did those areas require improvement?
3. What would you do to improve those areas?
4. What research would you draw on?

A model answer is provided at the end of this chapter.

What is not a QI?

Before moving on, it is important to understand what is *not* a QI. In healthcare practice we undertake a number of processes that evaluate the effectiveness of quality care such as audits, reviews and research studies; these should not be confused with a QI. Audits focus on ensuring adherence to regulations or standards without a plan to implement change – for example, compliance checks for hand hygiene without subsequent interventions would not be a QI project. Research studies seek to generate new knowledge or test theory, whereas a QI project focuses on improving existing processes based on current knowledge. Throughout your nurse training, you will gain experience in observing audits in clinical practice and reading research to support your learning. However, an audit, research, or review is not a QI project if it does not include a systematic approach to identifying problems, implementing changes and measuring outcomes with the goal of improving the quality of care. When you undertake a QI proposal as a student you will be putting forward a plan for change, to help improve the quality of care.

Activity 4.3   Reflection

After reading the section on 'What is not a QI?', reflect on any activities you observed during your placement that involved evaluating patient care. Why might these not be classified as QI initiatives?

A model answer is provided at the end of the chapter.

Importance of QI in healthcare

Having considered the definition of QI, and reflecting on your own experience of patient care, the next stage is to consider why QI is important. We know that QI helps to improve healthcare practices and patient outcomes – but does the NHS and wider healthcare sector require improvement?

There have been several reports published year on year about the substandard care provided within the healthcare sector. One such report was the Francis Report on Mid Staffordshire NHS Trust, which states:

> there needs to be a relentless focus on the patient's interests and the obligation to keep patients safe and protected from substandard care. This means that the patient must be first in everything that is done: there must be no tolerance of substandard care; frontline staff must be empowered with responsibility and freedom to act in this way under strong and stable leadership in stable organisations.
>
> (Powell, 2013, p. 66)

More recently, the Lord Darzi's *Independent Investigation on the National Health Service in England* (2024) highlighted that the NHS is in a critical condition – understaffed and underfunded, with a number of staff within the NHS becoming disengaged post-pandemic. Darzi also noted that the Care Quality Commission (CQC), which inspects the NHS, is not fit for purpose. As Lord Darzi (2024) explained: 'everyone knows that the health service is in trouble and that NHS staff are doing their best to cope with the enormous challenges. The sheer scope of issues facing the health service, however, has been hard to quantify or articulate'. The findings of this investigation are alarming, but also bring to light the need for QI more than ever. As a student nurse, you will learn about incidents of poor care and decline in patient safety; however, the opportunity to engage in and develop a QI will ensure you are equipped to guarantee safe care is always in place.

Undertaking a QI is not a linear process: it is one that requires careful consideration and the implementation of a rigorous process which we will be begin to discuss in the next section.

Principles of QI

The Health Foundation (2021, p. 11) outlines five simple underlying principles for QI:

1. understand the problem – pay attention to the data and what the data tells you;
2. understand the processes within the organisation and consider if these systems can be simplified;
3. analyse the demand, capacity and flow of the service;
4. choose the tools required to bring about change including leadership, clinical engagement, skills development and staff and patient involvement;
5. evaluate and measure the impact of a change.

Case study: Samuel, third-year student nurse, part 2

After reviewing the literature and speaking to his lecturers, Samuel begins outlining a plan for his QI proposal. He starts with applying the principles outlined above by the Health Foundation (2024). He works through the principles as follows.

Topic: QI – Improve documentation of patient observations among nursing staff

Principle 1: Samuel looks at the incidence of poor documentation and identifies any trends in the data – for example, is the documentation of observations poor at certain times of the day or night? Is poor documentation associated with less-experienced nurses? This helps Samuel identify the need for this QI proposal.

Principle 2: Samuel reviews the trust policy for the documentation of patient observations in the NMC guidance on this, including the link to the NMC proficiencies.

Principle 3: Using the data from principle 1, Samuel is able to assess if poor documentation of observations is linked to increased workload, patient flow, or general 'busyness' of the clinical area.

Principle 4 and 5: As Samuel is only undertaking a QI project proposal, he does not need to consider principle 4 and 5; however, some considerations under these principles are provided here as examples. Samuel could consider including the wider nursing team, doctors, ward managers, the education team and patients. When considering how to evaluate the impact of his proposed QI, Samuel could write up an audit and do a comparison with audit results over time.

Several authors have published various principles for undertaking a QI, but these loosely all look the same and reflect a change model process of:

1. identify the problem;
2. look at the evidence;
3. review wider process that may have an influence;
4. build and engage a team;
5. evaluate the change.

Activity 4.4   Reflection

1. Using Samuel's case study as an example, reflect on a QI that you would like to propose.
2. How would you implement the principles of QI as outlined by the Health Foundation?

As this is a personal reflection, there is no model answer.

It is important to remember that when undertaking QI in healthcare the patient should always be at the centre. The next section will discuss approaches to QI that reflect underpinning theorical perspectives.

Approaches to QI

You will learn in class about the various approaches to undertaking a QI. Some of the most commonly cited within the literature are as follows.

1. **Plan-do-study-act (PDSA) cycle**

   Plan: identify an area for improvement, set objectives, and develop a plan for change

   Do: implement the change on a small scale

   Study: collect and analyse data to assess the impact of the change

   Act: based on the results, adopt, adapt or abandon the change and plan the next cycle

2. **Model for improvement**

   Combines the PDSA cycle with three key questions:
   - what are we trying to accomplish? (goal setting)
   - how will we know that a change is an improvement? (measurement)
   - what changes can we make that will result in improvement? (idea generation and testing)

3. **Six stigma (DMAIC framework)**

   Define: identify the problem and project goals

   Measure: collect data to establish baselines

   Analyse: identify root causes of defects or inefficiencies

   Improve: develop and implement solutions for improvement

   Control: maintain the improvements and monitor the process

4. **Lean**

   Focus on eliminating waste and optimising processes to deliver more value to customers. Tools include:

   Value stream mapping: visual representation of all steps in a process to identify waster

   Sort, set in order, shine, standardise, sustain: organisational tool to improve workplace efficiency

   Kaizen: continuous, incremental improvements involving all employees.

   (Health Foundation, 2021; Institute for Healthcare Improvement, 2024)

There are numerous other approaches, each having their own strengths and often selected based on the specific context, goals and resources available. Often organisations may use a combination of approaches to effectively achieve their improvements goals. For this chapter, and to support you with undertaking your QI proposal, the focus will be on the *model for improvement and PDSA* cycle.

Model for improvement and PDSA

The model for improvement sets out three fundamental questions to help you begin your project; PDSA is then applied continuously as you work through your QI proposal. The Institute for Healthcare Improvement (2024) states that 'answering the three questions is an iterative process'; you will move back and forth between the questions and your thinking will likely change in answering each question as your move through the PDSA cycle. Figure 4.1 shows the model for improvement and PDSA as a continuous process.

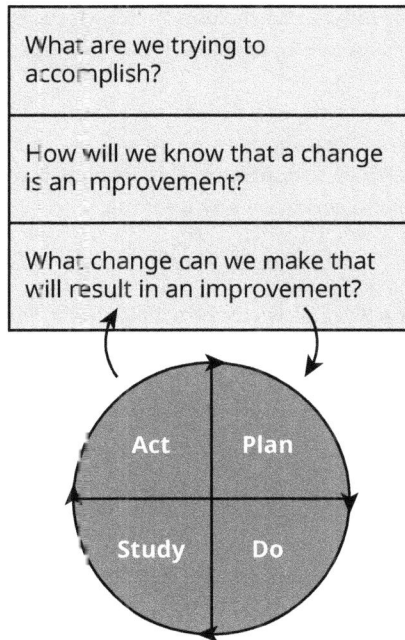

Figure 4.1 The model for improvement and PDSA (adapted from Langley et al., 2009, cited in Institute for Healthcare Improvement, 2024)

Now let's look at how to approach each question of the model for improvement.

1. **What are we trying to accomplish?**
   - This question is all about the aim of the project.
   - What are you improving?
   - What time/date do you want the improvement?
   - Looks at specific patient population – whose lives will be improved by this specific QI?
   - Where will the QI be undertaken – for example, is it within a hospital setting?
   - Who will you involve at this stage? It is important to consult those who are to set to benefit from this improvement when setting a clear aim.

2. **How will we know that a change is an improvement?**
   - How will you measure if the change has led to an improvement?
   - This might be in the form or an audit or survey.
   - This is a critical part of the process; you must be able to measure if the change has made a measurable improvement.

3. **What change can we make that will result in an improvement?**
   - What are your ideas for change?
   - Has this idea come from experience? For example, as a student you may have an idea on how to change an area in practice that you have seen while on placement.

- You will need to include several stakeholders in this – for example, patients and their family.
- You will look at best practices – for example, newly published guidelines and research.

4. **PDSA cycle**

- After you have addressed the above three questions from the model for improvement, you will then use the PDSA to continuously test your change, by planning, trying, reviewing the results and acting on any learning.

(Institute for Healthcare Improvement, 2024)

Let's re-look at the case study on Samuel, where he utilises the model for improvement and PDSA for his QI proposal.

Case study: Samuel, third-year student nurse, part 3

After learning about the model for improvement and PDSA, Samuel worked through his QI using the following approach.

1. **What am I trying to accomplish?**

   Improve the documentation of patients' six physiology observations (heart rate, blood pressure, respiratory rate, saturations, temperature, urine output) in line with local policy and the NMC by December 2024.

2. **How will I know that a change is an improvement?**

   Complete two weekly documentation audits to measure improvement.

3. **What changes can I make that will result in an improvement?**

   Samuel reviewed the literature surrounding the documentation of observations and found that this is an ongoing issue within healthcare. Samuel will carry out training to educate staff on the ward area. Samuel will print posters for the wards to help raise awareness of the importance of documenting observations.

Following this Samuel will continue to use the PDSA cycle to evaluate the impact of his purpose change and make changes where appropriate. The next activity will further support you in applying the model for improvement and PDSA cycle.

Activity 4.5   Reflection

Using Samuel's case study as an example, reflect on the model for improvement's three questions and consider how you would answer these in relation to your own QI proposal, chosen after undertaking Activity 4.4.

As this is a personal reflection, there is no model answer.

Understanding how to undertake a QI is the first step for you as a student; the next step is to structure the writing up of a QI proposal for assessment purposes.

Undertaking a QI assessment

Having used the model for improvement and PDSA, the next step is to write this up for your assessment. This section offers a general structure for writing a QI proposal, but be sure to follow any specific guidelines provided by your lecturer if applicable. For this section we will focus on Samuel's QI proposal which was to improve the documentation of nursing observations.

Abstract

- Begin with an abstract – a brief summary of your QI.
- An abstract aims to give the reader a brief insight into your QI proposal.
- Example: *This QI project aimed to enhance the documentation of nursing observations to improve patient care and safety. Poorly documented or incomplete observations can lead to delays in identifying patient deterioration. Using the PDSA cycle, we implemented changes, including staff training on best practices, regular audits and feedback mechanisms. Baseline data was collected to identify gaps in compliance. After implementing the interventions, documentation accuracy and timeliness improved by 25 per cent over three months. Ongoing monitoring and additional training will be essential to sustain these improvements, ensuring that patient observations are consistently and accurately documented.*

Background

- This is where you provide the background – what is the actual problem?
- Example: *Poor documentation of nursing observations poses significant risks in healthcare by compromising patient safety and care quality. Inaccurate or incomplete records can delay the recognition of patient deterioration, leading to missed or delayed interventions. This gap can increase the likelihood of adverse events, such as falls, infections, or even cardiac arrest. In addition, poor documentation affects communication between healthcare teams, disrupting continuity of care. Ensuring accurate and timely documentation is critical for patient outcomes, clinical decision-making and overall healthcare system efficiency.*

Literature review

- In this section you will provide a critical appraisal of the literature related to your identified QI proposal. You will learn how to undertake a literature review later, in Chapter 5, when discussing dissertation submissions.
- The literature you used within this section should give context as to, for example, why the documentation of nursing observations is a problem.
- Example: *XXXX (2024) highlights that poor documentation of nursing observations leads to delayed clinical interventions, miscommunication and compromised patient safety. XXXX (2021) identified that inadequate record-keeping increases the risk of adverse events and limits effective care coordination. Barriers include time constraints, workflow inefficiencies and lack of standardised documentation practices among healthcare staff.*

The QI proposal

- Here you will outline your approach to the QI proposal using the model for improvement and the PDSA cycle.
- Identify a clear aim.
- Set clear and specific goals.
- Identify the key stakeholders – for example, patients.
- Method – describe the changes you are planning to make.
- How will the proposed changes lead to an improvement?
- How are you planning to implement the proposed changes?
- How will you measure the effectiveness of the proposed changes?
- Ethics – identify if you require ethical approval; as you will only be asked to undertake a QI *proposal*, you will not require ethical approval, but you do need to make this clear in the write-up.
- Summary/conclusion of your QI proposal.

References

- You must ensure you provide an accurate reference list in line with your university's referencing system.

The above structure provides a starting point for you to begin your QI proposal write-up. While you may choose to structure your work differently, it's important to ensure all the outlined areas above are included.

Conclusion

This chapter began with an overview of QI in healthcare, explaining its core function as a systematic approach to enhancing patient care and outcomes. It emphasised the importance of QI in ensuring safety, efficiency and effectiveness within healthcare. The key principles of a QI, such as patient-centred, data-driven and continuous improvement were discussed. Moving on, various approaches for conducting a QI with a focus on the model for improvement and the plan-do-study-act (PDSA) cycle were discussed, offering practical insights for implementation. The chapter concluded with guidance on how to approach QI for assessment purposes, highlighting essential steps for successful QI proposal write-up.

Brief outline answers

Activity 4.1 Reflection

1. **Where could Samuel find out information on how to undertake a QI?**

He could first talk with this lecturer, who will be able to provide some context around what a QI is. He could also review the reading list given to him by his lecturer and access YouTube for helpful videos that discuss QI (some of which are provided in the annotated reading list at the end of this chapter).

2. **Who could Samuel speak with?**

His lecturers, student nursing colleagues or nurses within placement.

Activity 4.2 Critical thinking

Reflecting on your clinical placements consider the following questions.

1. **Did you see areas of practice which could be improved?**

Students often see areas in practice that require improvement, such as patient handover, waiting times, documentation. Noticing that an improvement is needed is not a criticism of care; as a student you are entering practice with up-to-date knowledge and can apply this to improving care.

2. **Why did those areas require improvement?**

You will apply guidelines and trust policies to patient care; it may be that the areas you see as requiring improvement are areas which are not working in line with policy or have outdated practice.

3. **What would you do to improve those areas?**

This is where you would apply the model for improvement and PDSA cycle.

4. **What research would you draw on?**

Up-to-date guidelines, literature, audits and feedback.

Activity 4.3 Reflection

After reading the section on 'What is not a QI?', reflect on any activities you observed during your placement that involved evaluating patient care. Why might these not be classified as QI initiatives?

Audits, routine patient care, routine documentation, administrative work, literature reviews, research, report writing and compliance checks – for example, checking the resus trolley equipment – are noted as ways to contribute to the improvement of patient care; they are not classed as QI initiatives.

Annotated further reading

Forde-Johnson, C, (2023a) *The Difference Between Research, QI, Service Evaluation and Audit in Healthcare.* Available at: https://youtu.be/_Rronp9X-Jc?si=CP2qILWWmEpExDVC

This presentation offers an overview of the difference between research, QI and service evaluation, giving practical examples and helpful tips.

Forde-Johnson, C. (2023b) *Plan-Do-Study-Act (PDSA) Cycle Example Using an Example QI Project.* Available at: https://youtu.be/6doaDaiWFwY?si=Pm9Ilq0Y_oDtMBHY

Excellent presentation giving an example of how to implement the PDSA cycle for QI.

Janes, G. and Delves-Yates, C. (2022) *QI in Nursing* (Transforming Nursing Practice Series). London: Sage.

This is an excellent book that drives further into QI, offering case studies and student-focused activities to support your learning.

NHS England and NHS Improvement (2024) *Online Library of Quality Service Improvement and Redesign Tools: Plan, Do, Study, Act (PDSA) Cycles and the Improvement Model.* Available at: https://aqua.nhs.uk/wp-content/uploads/2023/07/qsir-pdsa-cycles-model-for-improvement.pdf

This is a useful guide on how to use the PDSA cycle and model for improvement.

References

Backhouse, A. and Ogunlayi, F. (2020) Quality improvement into practice. *British Medical Journal*, 368, 1–6.

Health Foundation (2021) *Quality Improvement Made Simple: What Everyone Should Know About Health Care Quality Improvement.* Available at: www.health.org.uk/sites/default/files/upload/publications/2021/QualityImprovementMadeSimple.pdf. Accessed: 27 June 2025.

Institute for Healthcare Improvement (2024) *How to Improve: Model for Improvement.* Available at: www.ihi.org/resources/how-improve-model-improvement. Accessed: 27 June 2025.

King's Fund (2017) *Embedding a Culture of Quality Improvement.* Available at: https://assets.kingsfund.org.uk/f/256914/x/9fa0215ed8/embedding_culture_quality_improvement_2017.pdf. Accessed: 27 June 2025.

Langley, G.L., Moen, R., Nolan, K.M., Nolan, T.W., Norman, C.L. and Provost, L.P. (2009) *The Improvement Guide: A Practical Approach to Enhancing Organizational Performance.* 2nd Edition. San Francisco: Jossey-Bass.

Lord Darzi (2024) *Independent Investigation on the National Health Service in England.* Available at: https://assets.publishing.service.gov.uk/media/66f42ae630536cb92748271f/Lord-Darzi-Independent-Investigation-of-the-National-Health-Service-in-England-Updated-25-September.pdf. Accessed: 27 June 2025.

NHS England (2023) *Professional Nurse Advocate A-EQUIP Model: A Model of Clinical Supervision for Nurses.* Available at: www.england.nhs.uk/long-read/pna-equip-model-a-model-of-clinical-supervision-for-nurses/. Accessed: 27 June 2025.

NMC (2018) *Standards of Proficiency for Registered Nurses.* London: NMC. Available at: www.nmc.org.uk/globalassets/sitedocuments/standards/2024/standards-of-proficiency-for-nurses.pdf. Accessed: 26 June 2025.

Powell, T. (2013) *The Francis Report (Report of the Mid-Staffordshire NHS Foundation Trust Public Inquiry) and the Government's Response.* Available at: https://assets.publishing.service.gov.uk/media/5a7ba0faed915d13110607c8/0947.pdf. Accessed: 27 June 2025.

Dissertation (literature review)

Dr Phil Barter

Chapter aims

By the end of this chapter, you should be able to:

- explain what a dissertation is in terms of an assessment method;
- identify the different approaches to writing a dissertation;
- explain the purpose of each section within a dissertation;
- understand the methodological approach to undertaking a literature review.

Introduction

When you first started your nursing programme you were probably told about the importance of completing a dissertation as part of your nursing education. However, I don't think anyone would have mentioned that the requirements are often confusing and there are different types of dissertations. Understanding the requirements and the different types of dissertations will help you ensure you are on the right track with your own dissertation in your final year of your programme, where dissertation normally has a big impact on your final degree classification (Buckley, 2020). A dissertation can often be the accumulation of the skills and knowledge that you have learned through the duration of your degree programme, as suggested by Botten (2012). However, for a nursing student like yourself, the practice element of your programme is equally as important in your journey to becoming a fully qualified nurse, so your dissertation should show a link between your theoretical and practical knowledge. This chapter will start with a brief overview of what is meant by the word 'dissertation' and how it is used as an assessment method. The different approaches to writing a dissertation will be discussed, with a focus on understanding the process of undertaking a literature review-type dissertation.

What is a dissertation?

In simple terms, a *dissertation* is an opportunity for you to highlight your understanding of a specific area of interest within the field of nursing. By completing a dissertation on a topic of your choice, you can demonstrate your ability to research, identify different viewpoints and bring them together in a summary that could impact your future practice. It's important to note that a dissertation is not just another piece of work; it is a chance for you to demonstrate the knowledge and skills you have developed throughout your degree programme and highlight an area you are particularly passionate about in your nurse education. As a result, your dissertation is a crucial part of your academic and professional development in nursing. 'Thesis' and 'dissertation' are interchangeable words, used to describe the same piece of work – an *extended essay* or *report*. Through completion of your dissertation, you will demonstrate skills that align with the NMC proficiencies linked to critical thinking, research and evidence-based practice. This chapter will look at the different types of dissertations, before focusing on the typical format of dissertation used in nursing degrees as literature review dissertation, breaking down each section in detail so you have a clear guide on the requirements to complete your own dissertation.

Case study: Jasmin, third-year nursing student

Throughout the placements completed as part of her adult nursing degree, Jasmin has observed various levels of staff, on the different type of wards where she has completed hours. Jasmin has often reflected that these varying levels of staffing could have a significant impact on quality of care provided to patients. She hypothesises that wards with higher staff levels tend to offer more comprehensive and attentive care, while those with fewer staff may struggle to meet the needs of patients effectively. Jasmin is particularly interested in exploring the potential impact of staff levels on patient care for her dissertation. She believes that understanding this relationship could provide valuable insights into how staffing decisions affect patient outcomes and overall healthcare quality. However, Jasmin is finding it challenging to construct a precise title and research question for her dissertation.

Activity 5.1   Reflection

Consider Jasmin's case study.

1. Where could Jasmin seek support to help develop her research idea?
2. Can you suggest a research title for Jasmin's research dissertation?

A model answer is provided at the end of this chapter.

Different types of dissertations

Before we start to focus on the literature review dissertation and associated requirements, it is important, first, to outline the main types of dissertation you may see during your nursing programme. This will help you be clear as to which one you are undertaking. There are three main types of final-year dissertations which will briefly be outlined below.

Quality improvement project

As we learned in Chapter 4, a quality improvement (QI) project is classed as a form of dissertation that focuses on a problem, or solving an ongoing performance issue, with the aim of improving the quality of care. Typically, sections within a QI project will include objectives; data gathering; identification of performance; proposed solutions; implementation; and continuous monitoring plan. The QI will be linked to quality indicators to establish the degree of success of a QI. The linking to quality indicators enable the measurement of the extent to which the proposed QI plan has improved practice and patient outcomes. To complete a QI as part of your degree you would typically be given an outline of a problem and access to a data set associated with the problem – for example, a rise in pressure ulcers. The problem would be detailed in the form of a brief outlining the area of focus. From here, you would then need to analyse the problem and propose a possible solution. The format of a QI project is like that of a formal report. Further insights into the understanding of a QI can be found in Chapter 4.

Dissertation (primary research)

A *primary research* dissertation involves conducting original research to explore a specific question or hypothesis (theory): for example, does this type of treatment positively improve the health of patients? Primary research begins with a literature review to establish the context and identify gaps in existing knowledge. This is followed by a detailed plan (*methodology*) that explains the research tools you plan to use, such as questionnaires, tests and interventions. A description of how you would collect and analyse the data would come next. The central pillar of this type of dissertation is the establishment of new knowledge, or a different viewpoint on existing knowledge, which is demonstrated through the results and findings section. In these sections the data is presented and analysed to determine whether the initial theory is supported, or the research question is answered. Finally, the discussion and conclusion with this type of research will interpret the findings, discuss their implications and suggest potential further research that is needed and the impact on practice within nursing.

Dissertation (literature review)

This type of dissertation is known as a *secondary research* dissertation, or a type of literature review. A literature review-based dissertation is the typical format for final-year nursing students; you are most likely to be asked to complete one of these. Your lecturers will serve as supervisors, guiding you though the process of identifying a dissertation topic, developing your research proposal and addressing your research questions through the literature review.

To effectively complete this type of dissertation, you will need to follow these steps:

- identify a research question;
- decide on an approach to complete the search of the literature;
- use the results from the literature search to identify research papers that will inform the basis of your dissertation;
- the central pillar of this approach is to:
  o organise the literature into themes based on the papers you review
  o draw together the identified themes to form a cohesive viewpoint.

The overall viewpoint will then enable you to answer the research question you posed at the beginning of the dissertation. Furthermore, the findings will serve as a foundation for applying the results to clinical practice (Botten, 2012; Glasper and Rees, 2012; Jones, 2016; Karlsholm et al., 2024).

For the remainder of this chapter we will focus on undertaking a literature review, as it is the most usual dissertation format for nursing degree programmes in students' final year.

Literature review sections

A literature review can seem a daunting task, but, as with many assignments, once it is broken down into smaller piece it should become manageable and achievable. The first thing to understand about writing a literature review is that the sections are not completed in the same order as they will be presented in your final piece of work for submission (Buckley, 2020). Table 5.1 outlines the typical order in which the sections are completed, which will help guide your thought process through the writing of the dissertation. Following this, the rest of the chapter will address how to complete each section individually.

Table 5.1   Dissertation section writing order

Section number	Sections	Order of completion
	Abstract/ acknowledgement/ contents page	Last – this section is typically written once you have finished your review as it is a summary of the whole piece of work
1	Introduction	Fourth – normally you would assume that this section would come first. However, in writing up a dissertation this section is one of the last to be completed. The reason for this is that you will need to set the scene and describe the layout, which you likely will not be able to do until you know what each section will include
2	Literature review and methodology	First – this is the most important section and should be completed first, so you have an outline of the key themes which will be covered in your review; you will also establish your research question in this section
3–6	Themed chapters	Second – once you have completed the review of literature and identified the key themes, you can then start to write about the themes
7	Conclusions and application to practice	Third – once you have written about the themes, you will then be able to bring together your findings and answer your research question
	Bibliography/ references/ appendices	Fifth – this is an ongoing list, which should be maintained while writing and should contain all the papers cited and any additional reading completed which is not cited

Identifying a literature review question

Establishing your research question early in your writing will help you focus your searches for literature and then write the subsequent chapters. Your first attempt does not have to be the final question; you can always revise this at a later stage. You can use a method to develop your question such as show below.

1.   **P: patient, population, problem or disease**. Who are the patients, what is the problem, what is the population?

2. **I: intervention or issue.** Why are you concerned, what are they exposed to, what do you need to do to them?
3. **C: comparison intervention or issue.** What do we compare the intervention with?
4. **O: outcome.** What happens, what is the outcome?

If we use Jasmin's thoughts on her literature review, from Activity 5.1, we can identify the below:

1. P: adult patients;
2. I: staffing levels;
3. C: comparison of staffing level on different wards;
4. O: level of care given to patients.

Therefore, an initial research question for Jasmin could be:

How does the level of staffing impact patient care in adult nursing wards?

Literature review and methodology

Karlsholm et al. (2024) and Taylor (2014) suggest that the first part of a literature review dissertation should explain how you have chosen the journal articles to review. This includes identifying sources, setting criteria for what to include or exclude and detailing the search process, including the use of any software. Once you have established how you are going to choose your journal articles, you can then use a simple method as follows.

A simple literature review method

1. *Identify journals*: find journals and remove any duplicate articles.
2. *Assess articles*: check the remaining articles against the criteria for inclusion and exclude those that don't meet the criteria.
3. *Confirm list*: finalise a list of articles that are ready for the review stage of the dissertation.

At each stage of the literature review method you should keep notes as to how your list of sources was generated as well as why you also excluded papers. This will then provide your marker with justification for how you chose the final list of articles/sources used in your review.

The flow diagram in Figure 5.1 outlines the process for undertaking a literature review, including identifying and assessing literature from various databases and websites which you plan to use.

The process outlined in Figure 5.1 ensures that only relevant and high-quality studies are included in your dissertation while ensuring transparency and potentially facilitating others to reproduce the same results (PRISMA, 2020a). Once you have chosen a final list of articles, you can start to review them in relation to your chosen topic and research question. Buckley (2020) supports the notion that using a table to record the general themes for each of the articles, methods, sample population and findings will help you to keep your thoughts organised. Completing a review in this manner will then enable you to identify themes and discuss them easily in the relevant theme-based sections. Table 5.2 shows an example of this type of table.

Identification of sources for a literature review (N = the number of articles)		

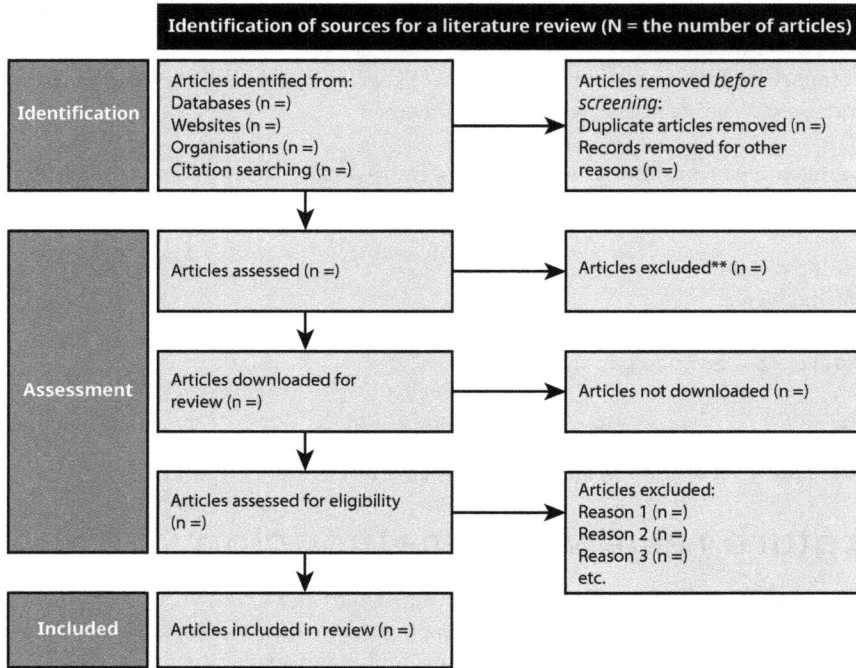

Identification

Articles identified from:
Databases (n =)
Websites (n =)
Organisations (n =)
Citation searching (n =)

Articles removed *before screening*:
Duplicate articles removed (n =)
Records removed for other reasons (n =)

Articles assessed (n =)

Articles excluded** (n =)

Assessment

Articles downloaded for review (n =)

Articles not downloaded (n =)

Articles assessed for eligibility (n =)

Articles excluded:
Reason 1 (n =)
Reason 2 (n =)
Reason 3 (n =)
etc.

Included

Articles included in review (n =)

Figure 5.1   Literature review process (adapted from PRISMA, 2020b)

Table 5.2   Example table record of literature search

Paper title	Publication year	Author(s)	Sample population	Methods (questionnaire)	Findings	Identified theme
Staffing levels in adult nursing	2024	J. Blogs	Adult	Data analysis	The level of staffing changed at night-time	Night-time staff levels

Activity 5.2   Reflection

Using Jasmin's research idea from Activity 5.1 (model answer at the end of the chapter), answer the following questions:

1. What words or terms do you think will be important in the search for literature to review?
2. As Jasmin would like to use the findings in practice, what would be the earliest publication date for the literature?
3. Do you think there are any other key items that are important to include in searching for information about UK nursing practice?

A model answer is provided at the end of this chapter.

How to identify your themes

After beginning your literature search, use your log (such as the example shown in Table 5.2) to identify common themes across the papers you've found. Once you've gathered a selection of journal articles or reports, use your log to determine which papers relate to which themes.

After identifying these themes through your reading, group the papers accordingly. Each theme should become a separate section in your dissertation. Within each section, critically analyse the papers based on the theme they represent.

A helpful way to structure each theme section is by following the approach shown in Figure 5.2. Start from the outer circle and work your way to the core, moving from the introduction to the conclusion of the section (Taylor, 2014).

For example, using the model answers from Activities 5.1 and 5.2, some possible themes might include:

- the type of ward where the patient is admitted;
- staffing levels;
- the time of day and how these effects staffing levels;
- the city or trust the hospital is located.

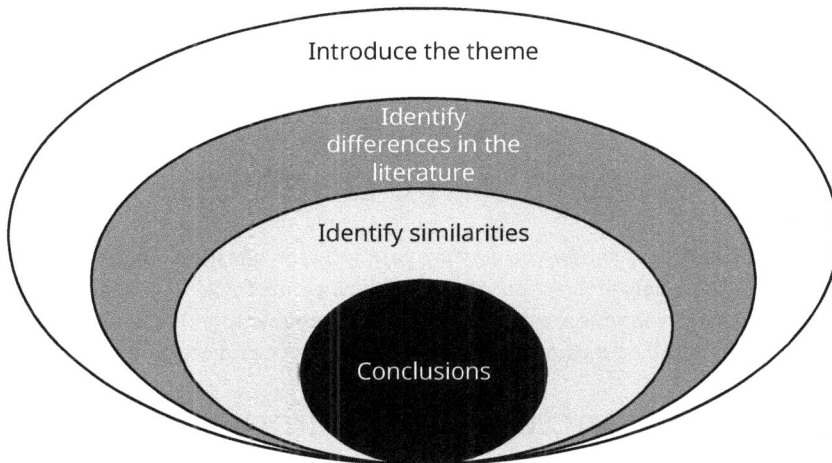

Figure 5.2   Writing about a theme for a literature review (adapted from PRISMA, 2020b)

Writing your themed sections

You are now ready to start to write your themed sections. The stages described below should help guide you in writing a section for each of the themes you identified using your literature search and log (see Table 5.2). You will need to follow stages 1–4 for each of your themes. So, using the examples in the bullet list above, you would complete the stages for *type of ward* and then again for *staffing level* and so on.

Stage 1: introduce the theme

Outlining the theme at the beginning of the section allows you to help your supervisor understand the boundaries of the theme, as well as the key authors and papers and the quality of the latter. Buckley (2021) notes that it is important to lead your supervisor through each section of your literature review in a systematic way. This will help the reader to understand your research topic and approach to answering the research question.

Stage 2: identify the differences

Identifying the differences between the papers, including population sampled, methods used and the findings, will help to establish which ones could be more relevant to the theme and answering your overall research questions.

Stage 3: identify the similarities

Having established the differences, you now need to look at the similarities between the literature found for the theme. This is a similar process to that for the differences, but looking for similarities in the papers: methods used, findings, population sampled, etc. Establishing similarities by using different methodologies increases the strength of those findings, raising the importance of the theme you have identified, so careful consideration should be given to this stage.

Stage 4: conclusions

The final part of writing about a theme is to identify the final positions and conclusions, having considered all the findings of the papers reviewed, including differences and similarities, through a critical prism. The overall conclusion for the theme will help you identify if the theme helps you answer your research question (Taylor, 2014).

Conclusion and introduction

The previous sections looked at how you develop your research question, find literature to answer that question and then analyse those papers to help answer it. Once you have completed those sections, you will start to see your literature review thesis coming together. It should be clear now what the themes of your dissertation are and how to introduce and conclude your dissertation.

Writing your conclusion and implications for practice section

The next section for you to complete is the conclusion and implications for practice section. The conclusion section has a purpose, which is to establish a clear message on the findings of your thesis and why the work you have completed is important. The purpose of the overall conclusion can be broken down as follows (Taylor, 2014):

- to answer your research question;
- to draw together the previous findings from the theme sections into one singular viewpoint as the established position of your dissertation;
- to indicate the limitations of your study;
- to identify further research that may be required;
- to explain how your findings could impact your practice.

Writing your introduction section

Once you have completed all the previously outlined sections, writing your introduction should be straightforward. This is because you should have a clear outline of the thesis and the main themes and points you have made throughout the previous sections. Therefore, in your introduction section of your literature review the aims and potential impact of the research should be outlined.

- Why do you want to complete this research project?
- How do you think it will impact your practice?

The introduction to your literature review should include a rationale of why the research needs to be completed, with a clear indication of the scope and limits of the literature review. The section should end with a suggestion regarding the methods used and an outline of your overall findings. The last part of the section needs to outline the main research question you are aiming to answer through the completion of the literature review.

Bibliography and reference sections

Once you've finished all the previous sections of your dissertation, the next step is to complete the bibliography and reference list. These are important because they show where you got your information from, allowing others to check your sources and better understand your ideas. They're also usually part of how your thesis is graded and they help you avoid plagiarism, which is when you use someone else's work without giving them credit.

A bibliography, on the one hand, includes any books, articles, or other sources you read while working on your dissertation, even if you didn't directly quote or cite them. A reference list, on the other hand, includes only the sources you cited in your writing.

Don't lose easy marks; make sure your bibliography and reference sections are correctly formatted. This can make a real difference to your final grade. Each university has its own referencing style, so check with your supervisor to make sure you're using the right one. Even small differences in citation style can matter, as shown in the example below.

- **Harvard**
  - Karlsholm, G., Strand, L.B., André, B. and Grønning, K. (2024) 'Learning evidence-based practice by writing the bachelor's thesis: A prospective cohort study in undergraduate nursing education', *Nurse education today*, 139, pp. 106239.

- **APA**
  - Karlsholm, G., Strand, L. B., André, B., & Grønning, K. (2024). Learning evidence-based practice by writing the bachelor's thesis: A prospective cohort study in undergraduate nursing education. *Nurse Education Today, 139*, pp. 106239.

However minor, the reference method changes the way in which you reference your sources and needs to be in line with the marking criteria. Ensuring this will mean you will not lose simple marks when your work is being graded.

A note on appendices

Your appendices normally contain supplementary information that is relevant, but not essential to the main work you have completed. This can often be further analysis you have completed of the literature which does not aid in the flow of a section, so was not included in the main body of your work. Any information included in the appendices needs to be fully labelled and cited within the dissertation; if it is not cited, then, generally, it should not be included in the appendices (Botten, 2012; Glasper and Rees, 2012; Jones, 2016).

The abstract

The abstract is the final piece of substantive writing you will complete for your dissertation. The paragraph should be no more than 250 words and be a summary of your whole dissertation.

Writing your abstract

This should mention each section of the literature review, starting with one line about the introduction, including your research question. There need to be a couple of lines on the methods you have chosen, which are often referenced to help with reducing the words used. The themes chapters should be briefly included and your overall findings in relation to your research question. The largest number of words should be given to the findings and conclusions of the paper. Once you have completed your abstract, make sure to read it through and check that it gives a full picture of your dissertation. It should help draw the reader in and make them want to read your work (Botten, 2012; Glasper and Rees, 2012; Jones, 2016).

Here's a simple structure you can follow:

1. **Step 1: Introduction (1–2 sentences)**

   • What is your chosen subject and why is it important to the field of nursing?

2. **Step 2: Aim of research question (1 sentence)**

   • What was your research question?

3. **Step 3: Methods (1–2 sentences)**

   • How did you identify the papers and sources you used to answer your research question?

4. **Steps 4: Research themes (2–3 sentences)**

   • What were the key themes you found through your literature review?

5. **Conclusion and implications for practice (1–2 sentences)**

   • What do your findings mean and what could be the impact on nursing practice?

If we take Jasmin's research idea (see Activities 5.1 and 5.2) and her research question of: *How does the level of staffing impact patient care in adult nursing wards?* using the steps outlined above this would then develop into an abstract like this:

[Introduction] The level of care in adult nursing is continually under the microscope and one of the elements which impact this is staffing levels.

[Research question] In this literature review, I aimed to answer the research question: how does the level of staffing impact patient care in adult nursing wards?

[Methods] The literature was found using the PRISMA method. Over 2,000 literature papers were found and, using an inclusion criterion of: publication year, UK-based literature and adult nursing, this was reduced to 200 sources.

[Research themes] From the literature the following themes were established: time of day, type of ward and hospital location.

[Conclusions and implications for practice] Analysis suggested that the level of patient care is impacted by staffing level, particularly during after-hours periods, and also that

this varied depending on the size and location of the hospital. I was therefore able to answer my research question and take this into my practice as I am more aware of the importance of care when I am completing after-hours shifts.

(*Note*: In the final version you generally do not use subheadings in the abstract.)

Activity 5.3   Reflection

Using an essay or scientific report you have previously completed in your studies, write a mock abstract of no more than 200 words to summarise your work.

You should try and include elements from your introduction, the main body and the conclusion, so the reader will understand the main message you presented in the essay in line with the steps used in the above example.

A model answer is provided at the end of this chapter.

Tips for working on your dissertation

Below are my top five tips for writing your literature review dissertation. These are just a guide and by no means an exhaustive list; you might wish to add some of your own and adapt them to the way in which you learn and have completed your assignments to date (Buckley, 2020, 2021).

1. *Plan your deadlines*: find out when your dissertation is due and any section submission deadlines and plan backwards from those points. You will then be able to identify periods which will be busier in relation to your other assignment work and those in which you will have more time to write the chapters. The ability to manage your time is also a key skill to develop through the completion of your dissertation and into your professional career. You might also want to use a Gantt chart to help with this planning (see Table 5.3).

Table 5.3   A Gantt chart example

Section/work	Months/weeks/dates
Literature review and methodology	
Themed chapters	
Conclusions and application to practice	
Introduction	
Bibliography/reference/appendices	
Abstract/acknowledgement/contents page	
Final submission	

2. *Choose a reference system*: RefWorks™, Mendeley™ and the sources manager in Microsoft Word™ are good examples of reference managers. Most institutions now provide access to a type of manager; if not. Word a has a built-in version. Managing the sources and references used in a literature review dissertation is a critical and often overlooked part of writing your thesis. A good reference manager will enable you to store all the

references you have found through your literature identification process; it will help you then identify which ones you have cited and which ones you have just read through (to be used in the bibliography). The final element that the package will support you with is to format the citations correctly, so you just need to copy these into the final dissertation. The set-up of a system might take some time, but this should be done at the beginning, so you don't have to repeat any search completed. Most systems also offer links to your university library and databases, such as Google Scholar, so the papers will automatically appear in the system ready for your use in your writing.

3. *Identify writing time*: the Gannt chart above (Table 5.3) will help you to identify writing time. Through your degree programme to date, you will have learned when the best time is for you to complete your assignments; you need to plan the best time in the day and week to read and then write the sections for your dissertation. You will also need to build in time to proofread and revise sections once you have received feedback from your supervisor; again, using a Gannt chart will help you.

4. *Confirm supervisor communication*: working with your supervisor in a positive manner will be key to the development of your ideas for your dissertation. Establishing how best to contact your supervisor and when you can expect a response is critical to ensure both your supervisor's and your own expectations are met.

5. *Identify a proofreader*: when you have completed your writing, it is a good idea to ask a peer support group, friend, or family member to read through your work to help with the flow of the work. The person you identify will not have seen the work before, so will be an 'outsider' and able to offer appropriate feedback and suggestions to help with the final draft of the work. Often when you have been working on a piece of work for a while, you will not be able to see some of the obvious changes that need to be made; therefore, a proofreader will be able to help with this.

Conclusion

The current chapter has provided you with a guide to writing your dissertation as part of your nursing education degree. By following the guidance provided here, along with the advice from your supervisor, you should have the knowledge needed to produce a dissertation that meets academic standards and contributes valuable insights to nursing practice. The type of dissertation will normally be pre-selected by your degree programme design, but knowing the different types will help you develop a greater understanding of the way in which research can be completed in other formats. The ability to use various sources of information and analysis to develop your argument is a key skill which will be crucial for your success in both academic and professional settings in terms of evidence-based decision-making; this is fundamental in the writing of a dissertation. As you reach the end of this chapter, let's summarise the journey we've taken through the different elements and things to consider to complete your dissertation:

*   *understanding a dissertation*: we started by defining what a dissertation is and its significance in your nursing programme. We discussed how it helps you meet NMC standards and prepares you for the challenges you'll face as a qualified nurse;
*   *types of dissertations*: we explored different types of dissertations, focusing on literature review-based dissertations, which are the primary format used in nursing programmes. This type of dissertation uses a structured approach to find and synthesise literature into themes, providing new insights into an area of interest;
*   *structure breakdown*: we broke down the structure of a literature review dissertation into manageable chunks. We suggested a non-linear order to complete each section, helping you develop your arguments and answer your research question effectively;

- *organising and critiquing journals*: we outlined how to organise the journals you find into themes and critique them to identify differences and similarities. This will help you formulate and synthesise a common viewpoint for each theme;
- *planning tips*: finally, we provided some top tips to help you plan your dissertation from the start, giving you the best opportunity to achieve the grade you are aiming for.

Remember, the skills you develop through this process will be invaluable in your future career, helping you become an evidence-based, competent and confident nurse.

Brief outline answers

Activity 5.1 Reflection

1. Where could Jasmin seek support to help develop her research idea?

Jasmin could seek support from her supervisor; the university study skills centre; and she could talk to her peers to help her develop her ideas and produce a title.

2. Can you suggest a research title for Jasmin's research dissertation?

A suggested title could be 'How do staffing levels effect patient care in a general ward?'

Activity 5.2 Reflection

Using Jasmin's research idea from Activity 5.1 (model answer at the end of the chapter), answer the following questions:

1. What words or terms do you think will be important in the search for literature to review?

Key terms could be: ward type, nursing staffing level, patient care, staff resources, patient type.

2. As Jasmin would like to use the findings in practice, what would be the earliest publication date for the literature?

A publication date range of the last ten years.

3. Do you think there are any other key items that are important to include in searching for information about UK nursing practice?

Other areas to consider: the time of day, the geographical location of the hospital, private or public hospital.

Activity 5.3 Reflection

As this activity will be unique to the piece of work, you should try and use this abstract structure:

Step 1: Introduction (1–2 sentences)

- What is your chosen subject and why is it important to the field of nursing?

Step 2: Aim or research question (1 sentence)

- What was your research question?

Step 3: Methods (1–2 sentences)

- How did you identify the papers and sources you used to answer your research question?

Steps 4: Research themes (2–3 sentences)

- What were the key themes you found through your literature review?

Conclusion and implications for practice (1–2 sentences)

- What do your findings mean and what could be the impact on nursing practice?

Annotated reading list

Buckley (2020), p. 2, *discusses how to achieve the best marks for your dissertation and links this to the Quality Assurance Agency (QAA) benchmarks for standards, which mention that the use of a rubric for this type of assignment will help you gain an understanding of what is being required from you in each section; also note that reading example pieces of previous dissertations will help you understand the outline and how the whole dissertation looks when finished. The two papers listed in this chapter by Buckley are excellent resources for writing a dissertation.*

Jaensson, M., Wätterbjörk, I., Isaksson, A.-K. and Falk-Brynhildsen, K. (2024), p. 4, *discuss the importance of agreeing your expectations with your supervisors and how this can help in the development of a positive experience in writing your thesis. Peer support is also mentioned here as a strength, which links to the points made in this chapter about the utilisation of friends or peers to help review and develop your work.*

Karlsholm, G., Strand, L.B., André, B. and Grønning, K. (2024), p. 5, *outlines that, while students' knowledge is supported by different types of dissertation, the literature review type is most popular in nursing education. The paper also features (p. 3) the use of a similar PRISMA process for literature search as outlined in this chapter.*

www.youtube.com/watch?v=TLvF8oWIXX8

This is a good video; it explains the key points of a systematic literature review, which form the basis of a literature review-based dissertation.

References

Botten, E.L. (2012) Writing your dissertation: where to start. *British Journal of Nursing*, 21(22), 1323 Available at: 10.12968/bjon.2012.21.22.1323.

Buckley, L.A. (2020) Planning and writing your dissertation literature review: a guide for final year degree veterinary nursing students (part one). *Veterinary Nursing Journal*, 35(9–12), 339–43. Available at: 10.1080/17415349.2020.1824141.

Buckley, L.A. (2021) Planning and writing your dissertation literature review: a guide for final year degree veterinary nursing students (part two). *Veterinary Nursing Journal*, 36(1), 36–42. Available at: 10.1080/17415349.2020.1841593.

Glasper, E.A. and Rees, C. (2012) *How to Write Your Nursing Dissertation.* Chichester, West Sussex: Wiley-Blackwell.

Jaensson, M., Wätterbjörk, I., Isaksson, A.-K. and Falk-Brynhildsen, K. (2024) Nursing students' expectations of group supervision while writing a bachelor thesis: a pre-post survey. *Nurse Education Today,* 139, 106257. Available at: 10.1016/j.nedt.2024.106257.

Jones, P. (2016) Writing your dissertation: a survival guide. *British Journal of Nursing,* 25(19), 1044. Available at: 10.12968/bjon.2016.25.19.1044.

Karlsholm, G., Strand, L.B., André, B. and Grønning, K. (2024) Learning evidence-based practice by writing the bachelor's thesis: a prospective cohort study in undergraduate nursing education. *Nurse Education Today,* 139, 106239. Available at: 10.1016/j.nedt.2024.106239.

PRISMA (2020a) *Prisma Statement.* Available at: www.prisma-statement.org/. Accessed: 30 June 2025.

PRISMA (2020b) *Prisma Flow Diagrams.* Available at: www.prisma-statement.org/prisma-2020-flow-diagram. Accessed: 30 June 2025.

Taylor, D.B. (2014) *Writing Skills in Nursing and Healthcare: A Guide to Completing Successful Dissertations and Theses.* Los Angeles: Sage.

Observed structured clinical examination (OSCE)

Dr Phil Barter

Introduction

An OSCE, or observed structured clinical examination, is an assessment method typically used in nurse education. This assessment method is designed to standardise an approach to test your clinical competence. Typically, this type of assessment involves using actors or lifelike mannequins to simulate scenarios which reflect clinical practice. An OSCE will have several components, with each having a separate marking criterion to ensure that you are assessed against the module learning outcomes. The OSCE stations are centred around a range of scenarios that are mostly practical, with some skills-based assessment and written parts. The marking criteria will be very similar in all nursing education programmes and underpinned by the NMC to ensure there is a standardised level of competency being assessed within nurse education.

The different stations of an OSCE

The typical OSCE stations you might see are as follows:

- *Station 1*: assessment (assess the patient);
- *Station 2*: planning (plan for two problems identified in station 1);
- *Station 3*: implementation (act on the care plan);
- *Station 4*: evaluation (evaluation and handover to your assessor);

- *Station 5 and 6*: clinical skills (perform four skills from a check list of skills; they can be paired together);
- *Station 7 and 8*: clinical skills;
- *Station 9*: professional values (understand the professional values in a given scenario; you need to give details of your action in relation to this);
- *Station 10*: evidence-based practice (in a given scenario; you will need to use your relevant knowledge to describe this).

General tips for all OSCE stations

Before we start to look at the stations in more detail, here are some general tips to keep in mind. As you work through each station, be sure to take notes – this will help you successfully complete the task at each one (Cerna, 2023).

- Don't be worried about writing the notes down as you go, just explain to the patient that you're making an accurate record of the conversation and assessment. This is to ensure that you can plan their care appropriately to ensure their needs are met.
- Make sure that your notes are legible, logical and easy to understand as you will need to hand them to your lecturer later.
- When assessing the patient make sure you consider all elements of the patient – not just what they are saying to you, but also how they look.
- Make sure you note the physical signs as well as the information that they give you. This will ensure you gain a holistic viewpoint of the patient's potential conditions or issues.
- While dealing with the patient always remember your bedside manner.
- Conducting yourself in a professional manner during each station is an opportunity for you to show all your soft skills, as well as empathy towards your patient.
- You need to demonstrate that you are listening and that you understand the patient. By reflecting the conversation back to the patient at certain points you can confirm accuracy, as you would do on the ward.
- Once you have completed your assessment and written all your notes, double-check you haven't missed anything – as soon as you end that station you can't go back and ask any more questions.
- Finally, thank the patient for their time and explain that you will be back to them shortly with their individualised care plan.

This chapter will now explain the OSCE stations and provide tips on how to prepare and maximise your chances of success in each one.

Activity 6.1   Critical thinking

Using the skills listed below, try to rank them based on which you feel are your strongest and which ones you think need more improvement. These are some of the clinical skills which could form part of your OSCE, as per NMC (2024):

- temperature assessment;
- respiration rate check;
- heart rate monitoring;

- oxygen saturation observation;
- blood pressure assessment;
- urine output analysis.

1. How do you think you can get support to improve the lower-ranked skills?

A model answer is provided at the end of this chapter.

In this chapter we will focus on the most relevant stations to help you prepare for your OSCE from a non-clinical skills perspective. As such, this chapter will only cover the first four stations in detail and provide a brief summary of the requirements for stations 5–10.

Station 1: assessment

What is the station?

For station 1 you will need to prepare to assess a patient (played by an actor). You will be given a patient history card which will provide all the details that you require to understand the patient's needs and any potential issues you may need to investigate.

How long will you have?

You will have *20 minutes* to do a thorough assessment. Make sure you plan your time out accordingly.

What is required of you?

You will need to utilise the training you've covered through your programme to complete a range of initial assessments, including undertaking the patient's vital signs, so you can try to formulate an understanding of two nursing problems that the patient is presenting with.

You will need to record your findings on an observation chart which will help you start to prepare for the next station – planning care. It is important to utilise the full 20 minutes in this station to ensure you get as much information from the patient as possible.

Tips for success

- When assessing the patient, make sure you consider all the elements – not just what the patient is saying, but how they look. Noting the physical signs as well as the information that they give you ensures that you get a holistic view of their condition.
- Don't forget your bedside manner!
- You are in an examination, but how you talk to the patient is still important. Show all your soft skills and demonstrate listening, understanding and empathy. Explain your actions to the patient as you proceed. Reflect the conversation back to them at points, as you would do on the ward. When you've completed your assessment let the patient know what next steps will be.
- Once you have completed your assessment and clearly written all your notes, double-check you haven't missed anything – as soon as you end that station you can't go back and ask any more questions. If you are happy that you have completed the note-taking and identified the two nursing problems the patient is presenting with, conclude your assessment.

Station 2: planning

What is the station?

For station 2 you will need to plan care for the patient you assessed in the first station. You will be asked to identify two of the patient's nursing problems and develop a handwritten nursing care plan for each. In addition, you must complete a risk assessment and any necessary referrals (Cerna, 2023).

How long will you have?

You will have *14 minutes* to complete this station.

What is required of you?

1. *Select two nursing problems for the patient* that you identified in station 1.
2. *Handwrite two nursing care plans*, one for each nursing problem, adhering to record-keeping guidelines.
3. *Complete a risk assessment* of your proposed care plans.
4. *Identify and document any referrals* required as a result of your care plans.

Note on corrections: If you need to amend your handwritten plan, mark the correction clearly so the assessor can distinguish your valid entry from the original.

Standards and evidence

- All nursing interventions identified in your care plan must be *evidence-based*.
- Where possible, have key references memorised for quick recall (e.g. Caballero, 2012; Peate, 2019; Beltran et al., 2024).
- Ensure your documentation style, corrections and referrals strictly follow OSCE guidance given to you by your lecturer.

Tips for success

- *Use the SMART acronym* to structure each care plan:

  - *specific*: target one precise aspect of the patient's nursing problem
  - *measurable*: define how you will know the intervention has been effective
  - *achievable*: confirm the action can be completed within the plan's timeframe
  - *realistic*: ensure you have the resources and expertise to carry out the intervention
  - *timely*: specify when the intervention will occur or be completed.

- *Time management*: allocate a set amount of time to each section (care plans, risk assessment, referrals), then briefly review at the end.
- *Clarity of documentation*: write legibly, structure each plan under clear headings (e.g. Issue, Goal, Intervention, Evaluation) and date/sign each entry.
- *Evidence at hand*: jot down concise in-text references or mnemonic prompts to demonstrate evidence-based practice without slowing your writing.

Pass criteria

To pass this station, you must submit:

1. two fully developed SMART care plans (handwritten);
2. a corresponding risk assessment;

3. all required referrals documented;
4. ensure completeness, clarity and adherence to standards.

Station 3: implementation

Hopefully, by the time you reach this station you will have completed two stations and are in the flow of the OSCE. This station will focus specifically on medicine administration. You will start this station by reading the prescribed medication from the patient's drug chart (normally your lecturer would provide a pre-written drug chart). By completing this you will demonstrate that you understand the medication you're about to administer. Remember that you are being assessed, so it's important to clearly verbalise each step you take with administering any medication to the patient. You then need to update the documentation to ensure that the dosage you have given is recorded correctly and ready for handover (Cerna, 2023; Lim et al., 2023).

What is the station?

For station 3 you will perform drug administration on a mannequin, guided by the care plans you formulated in station 1 and 2, and the pre-written drug chart provided by your lecturer. You must demonstrate safe, accurate administration of medication in line with the Royal Pharmaceutical Society (RPS) (RPS and RCN, 2023).

How long will you have?

You will have *15 minutes* to complete this station.

What is required of you?

You need to:

1. *review your care plan* and the pre-written drug chart to identify which medications you need to administer;
2. *follow the NMC medicine administration procedure* (below), based on Royal Pharmaceutical Society guidance;
3. *demonstrate each step* clearly on the mannequin, narrating your checks and actions.

NMC medicine administration procedure

Before administering any medication, you must:

1. *confirm* the patient's identity;
2. *ensure the prescription* or administration instructions are legally compliant, clear and include necessary details like the name, form/route, strength and dose of the medication;
3. *confirm consent* with the patient;
4. *check for any allergies* or previous adverse drug reactions;
5. *follow the administration instructions*, including timing, frequency, route and start and end dates and as follows:
    A. report any uncertainties or ambiguities about the administration instructions to the prescribing doctor and pharmacist immediately
    B. double-check any calculations, ideally verified by a second person, and consult the doctor or pharmacist if you have any doubts;
6. *verify the identity* of the medicine and check its expiry date;

7. *ensure that specific storage* requirements are followed;
8. *confirm that the dose* has not been administered by someone else – known as double-checking.

Tips for success

- *Verbalise each check aloud* ('I am verifying patient identity ... I confirm no known allergies').
- *Use the* **six rights** *mnemonic*:

    1. right patient
    2. right drug
    3. right dose
    4. right route
    5. right time
    6. right documentation.

- *Keep your workspace organised,* prepare one medication at a time.
- *Demonstrate safe technique* (a-septic, correct drawing up of injectables, etc.).
- *Document immediately* on the patient's drug chart.

Pass criteria

You must successfully perform and verbalise all the above steps, accurately prepare and administer the medications and document in line with the RPS (RPS and RCN, 2023). Now let's look at practising a drug calculation.

Activity 6.2   Practice drug calculation

Look at Chapter 8 on written examples; using the formula provided, see if you can answer the following question:
   A patient is prescribed 32 units of insulin subcutaneously. Each 10mL vial has 100 units of insulin in 1mL.

1. How many mLs should you administer to achieve the prescribed dose?
2. What is the correct procedure that you need to follow to administer the prescribed insulin?

A model answer is provided at the end of the chapter.

The fourth OSCE station asks you to evaluate care – let's take a closer look.

Station 4: evaluation

What is the station?

In this final station you will hand over your patient to your lecturer (assessor). You must convey clearly what care you have delivered, the patient's status and what the next nurse needs to know.

How long will you have?

This station lasts *8 minutes.*

What is required of you?

You need to:

1. *receive any new patient update* from the assessor at the start;
2. *incorporate that update* into your handover narrative so it reflects the patient's current condition;
3. *use the SBAR framework* (situation – background – assessment – recommendations) to structure your handover, see Figure 6.1;
4. *communicate assertively and concisely,* ensuring that your assessor understands what's been done and what must happen next.

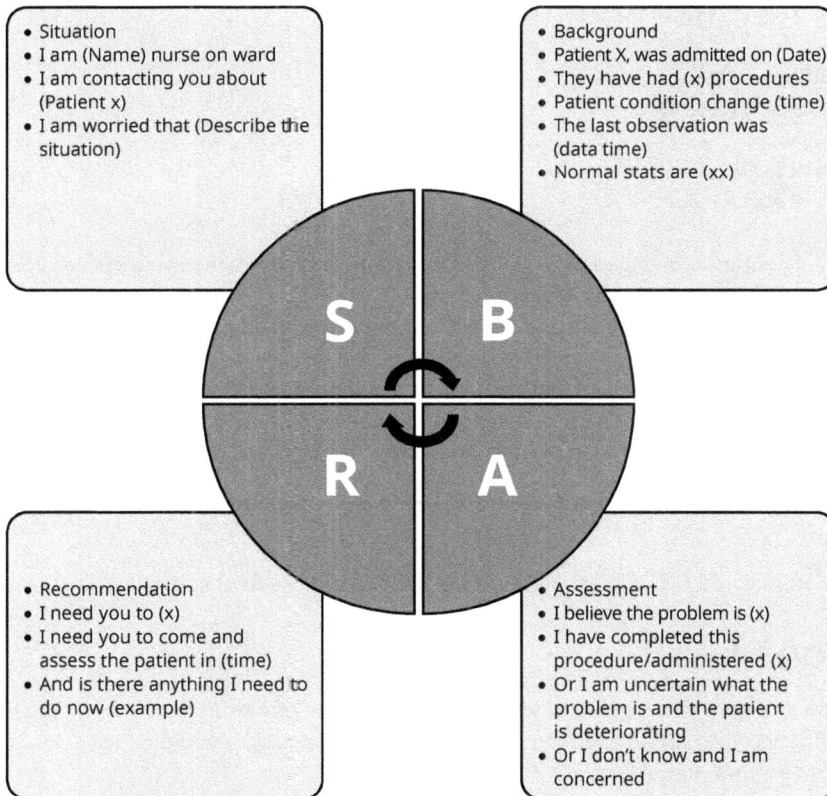

- Situation
- I am (Name) nurse on ward
- I am contacting you about (Patient x)
- I am worried that (Describe the situation)

- Background
- Patient X, was admitted on (Date)
- They have had (x) procedures
- Patient condition change (time)
- The last observation was (data time)
- Normal stats are (xx)

- Recommendation
- I need you to (x)
- I need you to come and assess the patient in (time)
- And is there anything I need to do now (example)

- Assessment
- I believe the problem is (x)
- I have completed this procedure/administered (x)
- Or I am uncertain what the problem is and the patient is deteriorating
- Or I don't know and I am concerned

Figure 6.1 SBAR (Park et al., 2019)

Tips for success

- *Speak clearly and confidently.*
- *Highlight critical information first* (e.g. 'Patient developed increased respiratory rate after medication').
- *Keep each SBAR section succinct:* aim for one or two sentences per bullet.
- *Verify understanding:* invite questions ('Do you have any questions about the plan?').
- *Document* a brief SBAR note if required, following NMC record standards.

Pass criteria

You must deliver a complete SBAR handover: accurately situating the case, summarising background, assessing the impact of your care and making clear recommendations for ongoing management.

Apart from handing over patient care, there are several other areas which you may be required to discuss during handover. For example, you may have spotted a drug area in the prescription or identified care which falls below the level of care expected. In handing these over, you will be asked to align your learning with the NMC Code (2018).

Activity 6.3   Reflection

Reflecting on any one of these scenarios:

- confidentiality
- professional conflict
- drug error
- possible abuse
- use of social media.

1. Briefly outline which part of the NMC Code (2018) would relate to your chosen scenario.
2. How could you check your answers?
3. Are there any other scenarios for which you think you could identify the relevant NMC Code (2018)?
4. Which scenarios do you feel you need to further revise in preparation for the OSCE?

As this is a personal reflection, no model answer is provided at the end of this chapter.

We have now covered OSCE stations 1–4, now let's look at the final stations 5–10.

Stations 5-10

The section will give you an idea of what to expect for the remaining stations of the OSCE; for further guidance you should speak to your lecturer and make sure you plan time accordingly to practise these components during your programme.

Table 6.1   OSCE Stations 5–10

Stations	Format and timing	Focus	Key actions and resources	Pass criteria
5–8: clinical skills	4 stations, each timed per skill	Fundamental nursing procedures and skills you have practised on placement	Review the marking criteria for each skill Practise under timed conditions Demonstrate each criterion clearly to the assessor	Successfully perform and verbalise four skills according to the marking criteria

Stations	Format and timing	Focus	Key actions and resources	Pass criteria
9: professional values	Scenario-based Q&A, 10 minutes, bullet-point response	Apply the NMC Code (2018) to an ethical/ professional scenario	Identify relevant code sections (NMC, 2018, e.g. confidentiality and professional boundaries) Write concise bullet points: action and code citation Refer to NMC marking criteria	Provide a code-aligned (NMC, 2018) response in bullet form that meets marking descriptors
10: evidence-based practice	Scenario + research article, 10 minutes' writing time	Apply given evidence (and your wider knowledge) to a clinical scenario	Practise reading a scenario and article quickly Bullet-point recommendations, citing the article and other key literature Practise concise, criterion-focused writing	Deliver focused, evidence-supported bullets that satisfy writing criteria

Tips for success

- *Know the marking criteria* for each station so you know what the assessors are looking for (for more information on marking criteria, please refer to Chapter 1).
- *Time yourself* in formative OSCEs to build confidence under pressure.
- *Use clear structure* (e.g. headings, bullets, SBAR) so assessors can follow your logic instantly.
- *Reference standards* (e.g. NMC Code, 2018; key literature) by author/year.
- *Reflect on practice*: after each mock, note any missed criterion and refine your technique or phrasing.

Why is the OSCE important?

We have explored the various stations involved in an OSCE, but why is this assessment important to you as a student nurse?

An OSCE allows you to demonstrate your clinical competence. The way the OSCE is designed is standard across all nursing programmes to ensure that every student nurse has the same opportunity to demonstrate their readiness for practice. The feedback you receive from the OSCE will aid you in your development and help you reflect on your strengths as a nurse and areas for improvement. The format of the assessment enables you to undertake the work in an objective manner, with bias minimised, so you receive a fair and transparent assessment on your readiness for clinical practice.

Activity 6.4   Reflection

1. Having gone through all the stations for the OSCE, how are you feeling about it?
2. Write down the stations which you are unsure about.
3. Where do you think you can find support for improving your ability in those stations?
4. Where are you studying?

Some tips on reflecting on the above questions are provided in the model answers at the end of this chapter.

Tips for working on your OSCE

Through this chapter we have now covered what an OSCE is, why it is important and the OSCE stations 1–10. Now that we've reached the end of the chapter, I'll finish by sharing some of my top tips for undertaking a successful OCSE. With all successful OSCEs preparation is key, so my top tips will help you focus on key areas to maximise your time.

1. *Practise, practise and then practise some more*

   - Regular practise is key, it helps to improve your competence in the essential skills required for the stations; rehearse the protocol required.
   - The use of AR or VR and simulation environments will provide an opportunity for you to practise a specific part of the OSCE in multiple scenarios to develop your mastery of the clinical skills in the same practice session.

2. *Good communication*

   - All the stations in the OSCE require you to effectively communicate to convey information to the assessor or the patient.
   - Communication skills to develop a rapport will be essential in several of the OSCE stations.
   - You need to make sure you always introduce yourself; when you speak to the patient address them by their name.
   - You need to make sure you act as though you are on a ward with patients.
   - When you are explaining your actions, you need to use clear and simple words to help the patient understand the outlined procedures and be prepared to repeat or re-explain yourself in a simpler manner.
   - Your ability to do this while displaying empathy will be critical to your success within the OSCE.

3. *Time management*

   - Remember the time limits for each station.
   - Plan and prepare to be able to complete the assessment in the time limit; there will not be any leeway given in the assessment.
   - Use a watch to help you manage your time; through practise try to plan the time so you can keep track of your progress through the station.
   - Practising all the stations under timed conditions, even the ones in which you are at a good level already, is important to give you confidence that you will be able to keep to time in the actual assessment.

4. *You are always being assessed*

   - You need to ensure you maintain your professionalism throughout the duration of the OSCE, even when not at a station.
   - You need to dress appropriately; be respectful of everyone involved in the assessment.
   - Adhere to the NMC Code (2018) and ensure your conduct is always ethical.
   - As noted in the communication tip, your ability to be empathetic with your patients while being polite and listening to their issues while recording relevant information is important.
   - Demonstrate professionalism throughout the OSCE.

5. *Reflect and learn*

- When you are practising for your OSCE, it is a good idea to reflect as it will enable you to plan your future practice sessions.
- Reflection allows you to self-assess and identify which elements you feel you did well and which parts you still feel need improvement to boost your confidence.
- Your reflection will also help you track the steps you took in your last practice, so you can pinpoint the areas you need to revise and don't repeat the same mistakes again, enabling new learning to take place.

Hopefully, these top five tips will help you develop your skills and techniques used for all the stations in the OSCE, which should lead to the outcome you are aiming for.

Conclusion

As you reach the end of this chapter, let's summarise the journey we have taken to break down each of the stations of the OSCE. At the start of the chapter, we began by defining what an OSCE is and its significance in your nursing programme. An OSCE is a mix of requirements which are designed to test your ability to demonstrate recall and use research, to critically analyse key information, develop a plan in response to the information, show your knowledge of the NMC Code (2018) and to show your practical abilities as a nurse through a variety of skills.

Throughout this chapter each of the stations included as part of your OSCE is outlined, with the key criteria you need to be aware of to be successful at that station. By following the suggestions made in this chapter, in addition to the guidance offered to you by your course tutors, you should have the knowledge you need to help you perform to the required level in your OSCE to enable you to demonstrate your ability to practise in nursing and operate confidently in an evidence-based manner as a nurse.

Brief outline answers

Activity 6.1 Critical thinking

Using the skills listed below, try to rank them based on which you feel are your strongest and which ones you think need more improvement. These are some of the clinical skills which could form part of your OSCE, as per NMC (2024):

- temperature assessment;
- respiration rate check;
- heart rate monitoring;
- oxygen saturation observation;
- blood pressure assessment;
- urine output analysis.

1. How do you think you can get support to improve the lower-ranked skills?

In the first instance it is always a good idea to speak with your lecturer. Take the opportunity to attend extra clinical skills teaching sessions, and continue to practise at home, in practice and with your peers. Review the resources that your lecturer has provided, and look at various other resources, such as videos, articles and books – this will help you in expanding your own knowledge and demonstrates that you have read around the topic.

Activity 6.2 Practice drug calculation

A patient is prescribed 32 units of insulin subcutaneously. Each 10mL vial has 100 units of insulin in 1mL.

1. How many mLs should you administer to achieve the prescribed dose?

The correct dosage is: 0.32 mL
(32 units ÷ 100 units) x 1 mL = 0.32 mL

2. What is the correct procedure that you need to follow to administer the prescribed insulin?

- *Confirm the patient's identity.*
- *Ensure the prescription or administration instructions are legally compliant, clear and include necessary details like the name, form/route, strength and dose of the medication.*
- *Confirm consent issues have been addressed.*
- *Check for any allergies or previous adverse drug reactions.*
- *Follow the administration instructions, including timing, frequency, route and start and end dates.*
- *Verify the identity of the medicine and check its expiry date.*
- *Ensure that specific storage requirements are followed.*
- *Confirm that the dose has not been administered by someone else.*

Activity 6.4 Reflection

No matter how you are feeling, it is important that you keep practising the OSCE skills that you are most unsure of, as well as revising areas you feel less confident in. This will help ensure you are well prepared and have the necessary knowledge to complete the OSCE components effectively. The annotated reading list (below) offers additional guidance; if you have formative OSCEs coming up, it is highly recommended that you take full advantage of these valuable opportunities.

Annotated reading list

www.youtube.com/watch?v=00pR5-taKiQ

This video on the NMC OSCE is a good resource for you, giving some great tips to start preparing from a regulations and professional body perspective.

www.youtube.com/watch?v=fh-kRKLoPPY

This video gives some more practical tips on your OSCE and is part of a wider series of information from nurse tutors which could complement the guidance and support offered by your course tutors.

www.youtube.com/watch?v=9innAlxKc-4

This video gives you some top tips to avoid anxiety on the day of your OSCE, so you might want to watch this in the days leading up to your OSCE date.

References

Beltran, C.P., Wilhite, J.A., Hayes, R.W., LoSchiavo, C., Crotty, K., Adams, J., Hauck, K., Crowe, R., Kudlowitz, D., Katz, K., Gillespie, C., Zabar, S. and Greene, R.E. (2024) Practice makes perfect: objective structured clinical examinations across the UME-to-GME continuum improve care of transgender simulated patients. *Journal Of Graduate Medical Education*, 16(2), 182–94. Available at: 10.4300/JGME-D-23-00573.1.

Caballero, C.A. (2012) *Nursing OSCEs: A Complete Guide to Exam Success.* Oxford: Oxford University Press.

Cerna, S. (2023) Components of objective structured clinical examination and its benefits, role and challenges. *Journal of Contemporary Medical Education*, 13(7), 1–2.

Lim, G.H.T., Gera, R.D., Hany Kamel, F., Thirupathirajan, V.A.R., Albani, S. and Chakrabarti, R. (2023) 'We need more practice': evaluating the role of virtual mock OSCEs in the undergraduate programme during the COVID pandemic. *Advances in Medical Education and Practice*, 14, 157.

NMC (2018) *The Code: Professional Standards of Practice and Behaviour for Nurses, Midwives and Nursing Associates.* London: NMC.

NMC (2024) *Test of Competence: Marking Criteria.* Available at: www.nmc.org.uk/globalassets/sitedocuments/registration/toc-materials-2024/marking/updated-rn1-adult-nursing-marking-criteria.pdf. Accessed: 4 January 2025.

Peate, I. (ed.) (2019) *Learning to Care: The Nursing Associate.* Edinburgh: Elsevier.

Park, L., Allan, J. and Hill, B. (2019) Data gathering and patient monitoring. In Peate, I. (ed.), *Learning to Care: The Nursing Associate.* Edinburgh: Elsevier.

Royal Pharmaceutical Society (RPS) and Royal College of Nursing (RCN) (2023) *Professional Guidance on the Administration of Medicines in Healthcare Settings.* Available at: www.rpharms.com/Portals/0/RPS%20document%20library/Open%20access/Professional%20standards/SSHM%20and%20Admin/Admin%20of%20Meds%20prof%20guidance.pdf. Accessed: 30 June 2025.

Chapter
7

Simulation and virtual reality

Cariona Flaherty

Chapter aims

By the end of this chapter you should be able to:

- discuss the role of simulation and virtual reality (VR) within nurse education;
- understand how to prepare for VR assessments within nurse education;
- differentiate between simulation and simulated practice learning;
- have an in-depth understanding of simulated practice learning assessment and its link to the NMC.

Introduction

Nurse education has adopted the use of simulation and VR as a teaching approach; it is shown to support students' learning and application of theory to practice. As the focus on digital literacy skills for student nurses grows alongside advancements in healthcare technology, the use of simulation and VR has become increasingly popular among both educators and students. Li et al. (2025) identified VR as a computer-based simulated environment where students can explore the virtual world. There are four main types of VR that you may encounter while undertaking your nurse training:

- desktop VR;
- immersive VR;
- augmented VR;
- distributed VR (Li et al., 2025).

We will discuss uses, as well as the pros and cons of each type of VR, later in this chapter. Aside from the use of VR, you will see simulation within nurse education being used to teach basic clinical skills such as cannulation and venepuncture. The NMC (2024) advocates for the use of simulated practice learning (SPL) to account for placement hours within the new standards. The NMC (2024) noted that: 'Following an extensive review, we have now made this a permanent standard, allowing up to 600 hours of simulated practice learning within the 2,300 practice learning hours students must complete.' Simulation within nurse education is here to stay, meaning we must find a way to embrace technology in view of student and practice learning. This chapter will outline the role of VR and then simulation within nurse education and identify approaches to support you in preparing for simulated and VR-related assessments. Clarity on the difference between simulation and SPL will be provided, with links made to the NMC requirements and associated standards.

VR in nurse education

VR is an innovative technology that you will see being used across nurse education to provide immersive hands-on learning experiences to enhance your skills and confidence. Due to cost implications, desktop VR is most commonly used, with augmented and immersive VR gradually being introduced. VR within nursing education is used to improve clinical decision-making, critical thinking and problem-solving skills and, like simulation, support the development of these skills in a safe and controlled environment. VR presents complex, dynamic scenarios where the nurse must make rapid decisions. This encourages critical thinking and will help you to develop your clinical reasoning skills in a safe, but realistic environment. The benefits of using VR during your training are identified as:

1. flexibility and accessibility;
2. using diverse clinical scenarios/experiences;
3. psychological safety and promotion of autonomy;
4. promotion of digital skills.

Desktop VR

The first type of VR you may be introduced to during your nurse training is *desktop VR*. This is where VR programmes can be downloaded onto your own laptop or laptops within your university. For desktop VR you will need a laptop or computer screen, mouse and touchpad to interact with the virtual clinical environment.

A software commonly used across universities for health-related programmes is Oxford Medical Simulation™ (OMS). OMS is installed onto laptops, giving access to a range of clinical scenarios. You will be given multiple opportunities to work though the scenarios, with a focus on developing your ability to assess, plan and manage patient care. The scenarios used reflect care across the fields of nursing, and support you with developing a wide range of clinical and professional skills. The scenarios will be timed, which will test your ability to work at pace when caring for an acutely ill patient. At the end of the scenario you are given automated feedback and scored across all areas of patient care delivery. After receiving feedback, you will be given the opportunity to reflect or come together as a group with other students to work through a debrief. You can practise the scenarios individually or while working with a colleague, caring for a single patient or a group of patients. The overarching goal of VR is to allow you to continually practise and rehearse your clinical skills in a controlled and secure environment, where it is safe to make mistakes and then learn from them.

Immersive VR

Immersive VR complements desktop VR with the use of a headset, which turns your environment into a clinical setting – in other words, you feel as though you are in the room with the patient. The sounds you will hear mimic a clinical environment; you will interact with the patient and the healthcare team and work through scenarios to assess, plan and manage care in an immersive VR environment. Like simulation and desktop VR, immersive VR will help you to enhance your clinical skills, promoting critical thinking and building your confidence to care for a range of patients and illnesses – ultimately leading to you being more competent and well prepared for qualification. Other reasons why immersive VR is fundamental to you during your training include that it:

- provides a realistic experience without risk to patients;
- supports hands-on experience;
- gives an opportunity to have real-time feedback;
- enhances your learning and sense of belonging;
- exposes you to a variety of clinical scenarios;
- provides an opportunity for team-based learning.

Your lecturers will review your progress when undertaking VR simulations and work to tailor teaching around areas where you may require further support – for example, administration of medication. This works to support students' individual needs and improvement with academic assessments. The next section will provide insight into how you can start to prepare for undertaking VR assessments.

Augmented VR

Augmented VR is a fully immersive virtual learning environment that is enhanced by additional sensory and information elements to improve learning. For example, your lecturers may implement augmented VR when teaching you how to care for a patient in A&E; you will be fully immersed using a headset, the sounds from the A&E will mimic real life and the patient data will be provided via monitors. This type of VR enables students to consider what it would be like caring for patients in an environment that reflects the real world. For example, if using a scenario in an A&E department, the background noise would be staff talking, the patient talking, bleeping monitors, phones ringing, etc. This type of VR gives you an opportunity to become comfortable in clinical environments that may sound daunting to begin with. Augmented VR is also available via OMS and other platforms, and is increasingly part of nurse education. Although the use of augmented VR is expensive, the benefits, for the most part, outweigh the cost implications, thus you may begin to see augmented VR being used more frequently to support student learning and preparation for practice. Let's now look at distributed VR.

Distributed VR

Distributed VR is a type of VR that engages multiple learners at once, where the learning environment is shared. This type of VR is used to support the development of teamworking and clinical decision-making. For you as a student this type of VR is linked to developing your understanding of how to work within multidisciplinary teams. Distributed VR enables collaborative working; however, it is complex to manage and support students from multiple disciplines at the same time. Therefore, at present, this type of VR remains in the early stages within nurse education, but no doubt will become a common feature in nurse training in times to come.

Having looked at the various types of VR, use the following case study to begin thinking about how you might prepare for a VR-based assessment.

Case study: Sarah, first-year student nurse, part 1

Sarah is a first-year student nurse. She has been doing well with her assessments so far, demonstrating a strong understanding of theoretical concepts and practical skills. However, she has an upcoming VR assessment which is making her nervous. She has never worked with VR before and isn't sure what it will be like or how she should prepare. She is worried that she will be overwhelmed and that her stress might cause her to lose focus.

Activity 7.1   Reflection

Watch the following YouTube video to give you a quick insight into what OMS VR looks like:

> https://youtu.be/sOG1cVvHUXo?si=Vkma9CW4dqwo_Ace

Consider Sarah's case:

1.   How could Sarah start to prepare for her VR assessment?
2.   What is the key thing Sarah needs to do to ensure success with her VR assessment?

A model answer is provided at the end of this chapter.

Preparing for VR assessments

Preparing for your VR assessments requires a combination of technical readiness, familiarity with the scenario content and an understanding of how to approach clinical problem-solving in a virtual environment. The key is practice; you will be given multiple opportunities to use the software, learn with other students and gain support from your lecturers. Failure to practise, familiarise yourself with the equipment and the scenarios will result in your not being prepared for assessments using VR. Although the use of VR for assessments is relatively new to nursing, it is a modality which is here to stay. The following list provides a series of tips and ways to support you in preparing for VR assessments; it is not exhaustive, but offers a guide:

1.   *Familiarising yourself with the technology*

     It is essential that you gain experience with the VR technology used within your university. Attend the tutorial sessions which your lecturers lead and watch the tutorial videos made available via the VR software. Ensure you know how to work the VR headset (if used), and ensure you are comfortable navigating the virtual environment.

2. *Review the scenarios*

   As outlined previously, you will be given the opportunity to work through several clinical scenarios. For each scenario, review the learning objectives and guidelines/instructions provided by your lecturer, including information on the assessment criteria – for example, you may be marked on how you assess, manage and evaluate patient care. For each scenario, take time to familiarise yourself with the patient's diagnosis, clinical observations and administration of medication; also look at managing an emergency, such as cardiac arrest. The key here is that no scenario should be a surprise to you if you have taken the time to rehearse each scenario prior to undertaking your VR assessment.

3. *Apply theoretical knowledge*

   To be successful in a VR assessment, you will need to show your ability to apply your theorical knowledge to the patient scenario. For example, to safely care for a patient having an asthma attack, you will first need to understand the underpinning pathophysiology. If you know this, you will then be able to administer the correct care required – for example, the medication required. Part of this will include assessing your ability to make decisions based on best practice and clinical guidelines to demonstrate rationale for choice. Therefore, it is important that you study the taught content that underpins each of the scenarios and that you have a breath of understanding in relation to support evidence.

4. *Apply clinical skills*

   As well as the application of theoretical knowledge, you will also need to demonstrate clinical skills. These will include basic clinical skills such as undertaking clinical observations, but also communication skills, teamwork and reflection, and your ability to act quickly in managing acute illness.

5. *Learn from previous VR assessments*

   Use your formative (non-assessed attempts) to make mistakes and learn from them. Review where you went wrong, and the feedback given to you. Book a 1:1 with your lecturer to talk through your feedback and support you to be successful in future VR assessments.

6. *Time management*

   VR assessments will be undertaken within a specific time limit, typically 30 minutes. You must practise each scenario within the time limit and ensure you complete all requirements before it has been reached. This will demonstrate your ability to work quickly under time-pressured clinical situations, such as medical emergencies.

Summary:

1. *Familiarising yourself with the technology*
2. *Review the scenarios*
3. *Apply theoretical knowledge*
4. *Apply clinical skills*
5. *Learn from previous VR assessments*
6. *Time management.*

Activity 7.2   Critical thinking

Look at the VR scenarios you have completed within university and ask yourself the following questions:

1.   What theoretical knowledge was required?
2.   What clinical skills were being assessed?
3.   What areas did I perform well in?
4.   What areas do I need to improve?

As this is an individual activity, no model answer is provided at the end of this chapter.

Moving on, we will now look at the difference between simulation and SPL.

Simulation in nurse education

Throughout your nurse training, you will be taught using *simulation* in a variety of ways. Simulation may be used initially to teach you clinical skills, such as observations, catherisation or cannulation. Once you have completed the theoretical knowledge that underpins clinical skills, your lecturer will then run simulated patient scenarios which will give you the opportunity to apply those skills to patient care using high-, medium-, or low-fidelity mannequins. The difference between the variety levels of fidelity simulation is based on the technology that is used. For example, on the one hand, your lecturer may use basic mannequins that can undertake a small number of tasks – for example, a mannequin that can be cannulated. On the other hand, high-fidelity mannequins will be able to interact more with you – for example, the mannequin may be operated by your lecturer using a tablet to answer your questions, cough, or show signs of respiratory distress. Advanced high-fidelity mannequins can have a seizure, cardiac arrest or hypoglycaemic episode. Simulation advances also focus on preparing your soft skills such as communication, breaking bad news and reflection using role play and peer-to-peer learning and feedback.

The Council of Deans of Health (2024, p. 8) identified the following as the benefits of simulation for students in nursing:

• providing a safe and controlled environment where students can practise without adverse risk to patients;
• increase student's confidence and preparedness for practice;
• provides an enhanced learning experience;
• opportunity for students to apply theory to practice through hands-on experience.

Your experience with simulation during your training may include using it while undertaking clinical placements. Healthcare organisations are investing in simulation environments to provide an opportunity for students to learn in practice with other healthcare professionals – for example, simulated life-support training and responding to emergencies. Clinical education often supplements nurse education, providing additional simulated clinical skills training for students while on placement and often having simulated teams who carry out this teaching.

The variety of simulated learning you experience during your training will depend on the simulation facilities available within your university. Most universities are moving to invest more into creating fully immersive simulated learning environments that look identical to real-life clinical environments – all of which is to ensure you are prepared for your placements and can practise your skills in a safe and controlled setting.

Activity 7.3   Reflection

Reflecting on your experience using simulation, outline what are the:

1. benefits of using simulated learning?
2. challenges with using simulated learning?

A model answer is provided at the end of this chapter.

Let's take another look at Sarah, who is now in her second year and preparing to undertake an assessment using simulation.

Case study: Sarah, second-year student nurse, part 2

Sarah is now in the second year of her nurse training and her next module is *advanced clinical skills*. This module is designed to teach her advanced clinical skills, such as caring for a deteriorating patient. The module handbook states that the teaching of these advanced clinical skills will be in the simulated clinical skills classroom; simulated learning will be utilised to support the delivery of this module. Sarah has never heard of simulated learning and is nervous about undertaking this module.

Activity 7.4   Reflection

Consider Sarah's case study.

1. Who could Sarah speak to about her concerns?
2. Where could Sarah learn about how simulation can help her learning?

A model answer is provided at the end of this chapter.

Simulation versus SPL

Simulation and *simulated practice learning* (SPL) are often used interchangeably within nursing. However, changes in the use of SPL to support up to 600 hours towards the 2,300 practice hours required by the NMC (2018a) to qualify as a registered nurse have resulted in the need to clearly differentiate between simulation and SPL. On a basic level SPL differs in that it requires application of the *Standards for Student Supervision and Assessment* (SSSA, NMC, 2018b). The Council of Deans of Health (2024, p. 7) differentiate simulation and SPL as follows:

> *Simulation*: an artificial representation of a real-world practice scenario that supports student development and assessment through experiential learning, with the opportunity for repetition, feedback, evaluation and reflection. This can include both physical simulation (for example, using manikins) and virtual simulation (for example, using VR).

> *Simulated practice learning*: practice learning scenarios are replicated, supported and complemented through a wide variety of simulation approaches.

> Council of Deans of Health (2024, p. 7)

And for SPL this is underpinned by the SSSA (NMC, 2018b) defined as follows:

> *Standards for Student Supervision and Assessment (SSSA)*: NMC standards setting out the roles and responsibilities of practice supervisors, practice assessors and academic assessors. They also set out expectations for the learning, support and supervision of students in the practice environment. In addition, they specify how students should be assessed for theory and practice learning.

> Council of Deans of Health (2024, p. 7)

You will experience each form of simulation within your training and each method will contribute towards your 2,300 theory or practice hours (NMC, 2018a). Having addressed simulation in the previous sections, let's now look at SPL.

Let's take a final look at Sarah, who is now in her third year and is preparing to undertake a week of simulated practice learning.

Case study: Sarah, third-year student nurse, part 3

Sarah is now in her third year. She has successfully completed her previous placements in clinical settings, where she has developed a strong foundation in patient care, clinical skills and professional behaviour. The NMC has just introduced the use of SPL into the nursing curriculum; it can be used for up to 600 placement hours. The introduction of SPL offers a new and innovative way for Sarah to continue her learning and development, which she is excited about, but she is also unsure about the expectations for students undertaking this type of learning.

Activity 7.5   Reflection

Having just read about the differences between simulation and SPL, consider Sarah's final case study.

1. What are the key expectations for students undertaking SPL?
2. Take some time to reflect on the differences and how each applies to your training as a nurse.

A model answer is provided at the end of this chapter.

The NMC and SPL

In response to the COVID-19 pandemic, the NMC implemented the emergency standards which allow universities and their practice partners to deliver some practice learning using simulation. Following positive review of this, the NMC made this approach a permanent fixture where universities could run up to 600 hours of SPL. The NMC has outlined that SPL must do the following:

*   meet the *Standards for Pre-registration Nursing Programmes* (NMC, 2023) for practice learning;
*   meet the *Standards for Student Supervision and Assessment* (NMC, 2018b);
*   ensure those supervising simulated practice are appropriately prepared to do so (practice supervisors);
*   demonstrate achievement of the learning outcomes that would have been experienced in a practice setting;
*   be used to enhance practice learning:
    *   simulation provides opportunities to explore diverse areas of practice and experience situations less frequently encountered in the practice setting;
*   enable active engagement in practice learning:
    *   students need to learn to practise.

NMC (2024)

The NMC also clearly identifies what does *not* constitute simulation – for instance, learning that supports theoretical understanding, but lacks contextualisation or supervision, such as a lecture, is not considered simulation. The benefits of SPL which have not yet been mentioned are as follows:

*   *cultural competence*: exposure to caring for simulated scenarios from a diverse population, to support understanding of cultural issues within clinical practice;
*   *boosts confidence*: having the opportunity to practise and make errors in a safe environment will help you in becoming more confident in practice when providing patient care.

As a student, the number of SPL hours you can claim towards your 2,300 will depend on the number of hours your university has been approved to deliver. This will vary across universities depending on the facilities available, but a typical week of SPL may be delivered as follows:

- *day 1–4*: working on the clinical ward (within the university), you will be expected to arrive on time, have a handover and work with a group of students to care for four to six patients within a simulated ward area. Your lecturer will observe how you work and run simulated clinical problems to see how you perform – for example, they may simulate your patient having a hypoglycaemic episode. You will be expected to manage this, call for support and work as a team to manage the patient. Several universities also use actors to bring the SPL experience to life, observing your communication skills and how you respond to events – individually and as a group. This will normally end with a debrief where you will be given an opportunity to discuss your learning and reflections;
- *day 5*: you may work on a VR scenario, then attend an online briefing on how you worked through it where you provide the rationale for the care you provided. The lecturer will facilitate the discussion, which could involve peer and service user feedback.

The above is just an example; each university will have its own way of delivering SPL, but each way will be in line with the NMC's requirements as outlined previously.

Activity 7.6   Evidence-based assessment

Look at the NMC (2018a) *Standards of Proficiency for Registered Nurses* and answer the following question:

1.   What proficiencies could be assessed when undertaking SPL?

A model answer is provided at the end of this chapter.

Preparing for SPL assessments

Any SPL assessment will reflect the NMC (2018b) *Standards of Proficiency for Registered Nurses*. When it comes to SPL, as a student you will need to treat it as if you were in clinical practice, and you will be assessed as such. Focusing first on professional values, your lecturers will expect you to:

- arrive on time for the patient handover;
- arrive wearing your uniform in line with policy, including the correct footwear and showing an ID badge;
- if you are unwell, you will be expected to report your absence to your lecturer as you would if you were in clinical practice;
- use listening skills when attending the patient handover;
- use communication skills for a range of patient and clinical scenarios;

- use teamworking skills;
- demonstrate professionalism.

When caring for the simulated patients the following areas will be looked at in terms of assessment:

- your theoretical knowledge of range of patient illness and your clinical judgement and how you plan care;
- your ability to undertake a range of clinical skills, which may include observations, taking bloods, inserting catheter care and attending to patient's hygiene needs, as well as technical skills such as CPR;
- your knowledge of how to manage an emergency or deal with a complex or aggressive patient;
- how you respond to conflict within the team;
- how you break bad news to a patient, or give feedback to colleagues;
- infection control and risk management, including patient safety;
- ethical considerations such as consent;
- time management and organisation skills;
- health promotion and how you provide health-related education to your patient.

The above list is not exhaustive; the way you prepare for SPL assessments is in fact the same way in which you would prepare for clinical placements. This preparation will involve a combination of practical, academic and personal strategies to ensure your readiness for the practice expectations. Some of this preparation will be as follows.

Reviewing your theory

You must ensure you are up to date with your theoretical learning; this will include understanding clinical guidelines. Your lecturers will run SPL in line with up-to-date research and you will be expected to provide rationale for the care you administer to the simulated patient.

Prepare for clinical skills

Review the learning you have undertaken in relation to clinical skills. If you are unsure how to undertake a clinical skill, make sure you speak with your lecturer for extra support.

Familiarise yourself with the simulated clinical area

Take note of where things are placed – for example, the equipment, emergency call bell, fire exit, crash trolley and nurses' station.

Be open to feedback

You will receive feedback from your lecturers, peers and service users during your SPL, which provides a valuable way for you to develop the areas where you may require improvement, as well as understand your key strengths.

Understand reflection

A key aspect of SPL is that you are provided with an opportunity to reflect on learning and undertake a debrief. Your lecturers will be observing your ability to reflect on practice and on action – which is a fundamental nursing skill.

Understand the role of the practice assessor (PA), practice supervisor (PS) and academic assessor (AA)

The NMC identifies these three roles as follows:

- a *PA* assesses and confirms your achievement of learning outcomes set out for each of your practice learning experiences or placements. SPL is considered a placement because it contributed to your NMC hours. The NMC (2018b) states that the PA 'assesses the student's overall performance for their practice learning, taking account of whether or not the relevant proficiencies and programmes outcomes have been met, and if they display the required values of their professional role';
- a *PS* 'supports and supervises nursing and midwifery students' learning in the practice learning environment. All students must be supervised while learning in practice environments' (NMC, 2018b, p. 6);
- an *AA* is expected to 'collate' and 'confirm' the student's academic and practice learning outcomes for the part of the programme they are assigned to the student, before recommending them for progression on to the next part of the programme (NMC, 2018b).

It is important to understand that all the above roles can support you in achieving your SPL objectives. To summarise, your preparation for SPL assessment will include the following:

- alignment to the NMC (2018a) *Standards of Proficiency for Registered Nurses*;
- demonstration of professional values;
- reviewing your theory;
- preparation for clinical skills;
- familiarisation with the simulated clinical area;
- being open to feedback;
- understanding reflection;
- understanding the role of the PA, PS and AA.

Conclusion

This chapter has provided an outline of the essential roles that simulation and VR play within nurse education. Through simulation and VR, as a nursing student you will have the opportunity to engage in realistic, controlled scenarios that enhance both your clinical skills and decision-making abilities. The opportunity to practise in such environments will provide you with a deeper understanding of clinical procedures, fostering critical thinking and enabling you to develop the confidence needed to work within a range of healthcare settings. We examined how to prepare for VR assessments within nursing education, noting the importance of familiarity with the technology and the specific expectations of these assessments. Preparation for VR assessments includes knowing how to integrate the learning objectives of these virtual experiences with real-world nursing and the NMC professional standards.

This chapter provided insight into the difference between simulation and SPL. While both are valuable within nursing education, it is important to recognise that simulation focuses more on replicating specific clinical situations, whereas SPL involves a more rounded, immersive experience that reflects clinical practice learning. Furthermore, the chapter highlighted the link between SPL assessments and NMC standards. By aligning these, educators ensure that you, as a student, meet the regulatory requirements for safe and effective practice. Through careful preparation and adhering to professional standards, you will benefit greatly from the use of VR, simulation and SPL throughout your training.

Brief outline answers

Activity 7.1 Reflection

1. How could Sarah start to prepare for her VR assessment?

I would advise Sarah to speak with her lecturers, then read the assessment information provided such as the marking criteria/rubric (see Chapter 1 for more information on this). Sarah should also attend all practice sessions, where her lecturers will outline what to expect in the summative VR assessment.

2. What is the key thing Sarah needs to do to ensure success with her VR assessment?

Take her time, read the assessment criteria, understand what is being asked for in the VR assessment. Above all else, practise beforehand.

Activity 7.3 Reflection

1. What are the benefits of using simulated learning?

Simulated learning provides a safe learning environment for students to practise caring for a range of patients across different clinical settings. Students can safely make mistakes and learn from these to improve their practice when they are on placement.

2. What are the challenges with using simulated learning?

It requires students to learn how to use advanced technology, which can sometimes be daunting; however, lecturers are equipped to support students. Students will be working alongside their peers and may not be as confident to begin with, but, again, remember this is a safe and supportive learning environment.

Activity 7.4 Reflection

1. Who could Sarah speak to about this?

Sarah should speak with her lecturers; they will provide support and encouragement.

2. Where could Sarah learn about how simulation can help her learning?

The NMC provides student-friendly information on simulation; the reference for this website is in the annotated reading section.

Activity 7.5 Reflection

1. What are the key expectations for students undertaking SPL?

The key difference is that SPL is supervised in line with the SSSA standards and contributes towards practice learning hours. SPL, on the one hand, is contextualised learning, reflecting clinical practice. Simulation, on the other hand, is learning that is not supervised in line with the SSSA and is not contextualised to reflect practice learning.

2. Take some time to reflect on the differences and how each applies to your training as a nurse.

The expectations of students are the same as if you were attending clinical practice – for example, you must turn up on time, be in uniform, maintain professional values and contribute to patient care as set out by the lecturer.

Activity 7.6 Evidence-based assessment

1. What proficiencies could be assessed when undertaking SPL?

Professional values are continuously assessed regardless of the setting. Although specific proficiencies have not been mandated within SPL, your university will normally be able to provide information on this. Some universities may sign off several proficiencies, others may not; it very much depends on university.

Annotated further reading

NMC (2024) *Simulated Practice Learning.* Available at: www.nmc.org.uk/standards/ guidance/supporting-information-for-our-education-and-training-standards/simulated-practice-learning/

Referenced in this chapter, this website has lots of information on SPL.

RCN (2023) *Position on the use of Simulation-based Learning in Pre and Post Registration Education.* Available at: www.rcn.org.uk/About-us/Our-Influencing-work/Position-statements/rcn-position-statement-on-the-use-of-simulation-based-learning

This webpage provides an extensive and useful reference list to aid your learning on simulation-based learning.

References

Council of Deans of Health (2024) *Simulation in Nursing Education: An Evidence Base for the Future.* Available at: www.councilofdeans.org.uk/wp-content/uploads/2024/01/CoDH-ARU-Simulation-in-Nursing-Education-Report-Jan-2024.pdf. Accessed 2 July 2025.

Li, Y., Chen, Y., Wei, G., Ma, F., Hu, Q., Wei, W. and Bai, Y. (2025) Application of desktop virtual reality technology in nursing student education: a realist review. *BMC Medical Education*, 25(78), 1–17.

NMC (2018a) *Standards of Proficiency for Registered Nurses.* Available at: www.nmc.org. uk/globalassets/sitedocuments/standards/2024/standards-for-pre-registration-nursing-programmes.pdf. Accessed 2 July 2025.

NMC (2018b) *Standards for Student Supervision and Assessment.* Available at: www.nmc.org. uk/standards-for-education-and-training/standards-for-student-supervision-and-assessment/. Accessed 2 July 2025.

NMC (2023) *Standards for Pre-registration Nursing Programmes.* Available at: www.nmc.org. uk/globalassets/sitedocuments/standards/2024/standards-of-proficiency-for-nurses.pdf. Accessed 2 July 2025.

NMC (2024) *Simulated Practice Learning.* Available at: www.nmc.org.uk/standards/guidance/ supporting-information-for-our-education-and-training-standards/simulated-practice-learning/. Accessed 2 July 2025.

Chapter 8

Written exams: drug calculation

Cariona Flaherty

Chapter aims

By the end of this chapter you should be able to:

- understand the use of written exams as an assessment method within university and nurse education specifically;
- describe the various types of written exams used within nurse education;
- identify ways to succeed when undertaking the different types of written exams;
- have an in-depth understanding of undertaking a drug calculation exam and its link to practice and the NMC.

Introduction

Written exams are a fundamental component of undergraduate nurse education, used to assess your knowledge, comprehension and application of key concepts in nursing practice, theory and clinical skills. Some of the purposes of written exams within nurse education include:

- assessment of student knowledge;
- critical thinking;
- application to practice;
- evaluation of students' learning;
- evaluation of students' professional accountability.

In undergraduate nurse education, written exams also ensure you are meeting the standards set by the NMC. Specifically, the NMC *Standards of Proficiency for Registered Nurses* (2018) include the requirement that as a student nurse you must successfully complete a drug calculation exam with a 100 per cent pass mark to ensure competence in the safe administration of medication. Apart from the drug calculation exam, other forms of written exams that you might have may include:

- multiple-choice questions (MCQs);
- short-answer/essay question;
- case studies;
- true or false questions.

Although exams contribute to the assessment of knowledge, you may find exams stressful. Often exams do not reflect practice – therefore students tend to prefer alternative means of assessment, such as essays. Reasons you find exams stressful could include:

- *academic expectations*: your course will have challenging topics that increase in complexity as you move through the academic years. With this, you may find that exams become more challenging, and this can cause a degree of stress;
- *time limits*: undertaking an exam within a certain limit can be incredibly stressful; you may find it hard to concentrate on the exam itself;
- *lack of confidence*: if you are new to undertaking exams or have had negative experiences in the past, you may struggle with self-doubt and confidence.

However, as some exams are a requirement within nurse education, it is important that you understand how to prepare and succeed when undertaking written exams. This chapter will discuss the various types of written exams and will identify ways to help you succeed, with a focus on the drug calculation exam and how this links to the NMC and practice.

Case study: George, first-year student nurse, part 1

George is a mature student who decided to return to education after several years of working in a different field. The transition back to academic life has been challenging for George, as he has had to adapt to new study techniques and re-acquaint himself with the rigours of academic assessments. One of George's upcoming assessments is a written MCQ exam on anatomy and physiology. George has not undertaken an exam in a long time and is concerned about how he will remember the information needed to achieve a pass mark. George is also struggling with understanding the difference between an MCQ and other written exams.

Activity 8.1   Reflection

1. Consider George's case study. How could George begin preparing for his upcoming MCQ exam?
2. Who could George talk to about his concerns?

A model answer is provided at the end of this chapter.

Written exams

Undertaking exams can be stressful, as for George; often students find it hard to know how to begin studying. It is helpful to begin with an understanding of why you are being asked to complete assessments and written exams. Ortega-Sanchez (2016, p. 145) identified that 'the sole purpose of assessment tasks is to verify the students' achievement of the learning outcomes'. Learning outcomes are measurable skills or knowledge that you should be able to demonstrate after undertaking a learning or training experience. How learning outcomes are measured depends on the assessment task being used. For example, assessments may be in the form of a written essay, quality improvement (QI) project or a written exam. Whichever the assessment strategy, the purpose should be to provide you with an opportunity to demonstrate what you can do and what you know (Ortega-Sanchez, 2016). You may find that some exams are used in combination with other types of assessments – for example, an MCQ and a reflective essay. The reason for this is to assess your different levels of knowledge, with the MCQ assessing low-level knowledge such as remembering (although not always), and the reflective essay assessing higher levels of knowledge such as analyses or evaluation. In nursing, the various levels of knowledge being assessed will depend on the year of study you are in and the complexity of knowledge being assessed. For example, in the first year you will be learning about anatomy and physiology and, typically, this is assessed using an MCQ. In contrast, in the third year, you will be learning about complex pathophysiology and its application to patient care – using an MCQ may not reveal the level of knowledge required, therefore you may be expected to undertake a long-answer written exam using a case study. MCQs can also assess higher levels of knowledge, provided the questions are designed to evaluate advanced cognitive abilities (Leung et al., 2008). Now, let's look at some of the types of written exams you may encounter while undertaking your nurse training:

- MCQs
- open-book or closed-book (seen or unseen) written exam
- drug calculation.

MCQs

MCQs can be used to test a broad range of topics – not only recall of information, but also to test clinical reasoning and decision-making. MCQs consist of a series of questions or statements followed by several possible answers, which are often labelled as options or choices. Among these options, only one is the correct answer, while the other possible answers are used to distract and challenge your knowledge and understanding. MCQs can cover a wide range of topics within nursing, including anatomy and physiology, pathophysiology, nursing interviewing, pharmacology, patient assessment and legal/ethical issues. You will encounter several forms of MCQs – for example, short- or long-answer questions, labelling of diagrams and open- and closed-book MCQ (this will be discussed later). As well as the use of short answers, MCQs can be designed to test longer questions based on case studies, therefore providing you with the opportunity to highlight your ability to think critically. By designing well-structured questions, your lecturers can assess not only theoretical knowledge, but also your ability to make clinical decisions, prioritise care and solve problems that reflect clinical practice.

There are several advantages to using MCQ as an assessment method in nursing such as:

- *efficiency*: the nature of MCQs being quick, they support the assessment of a broad range of knowledge – for example, a first-year MCQ may be used to assess your understanding of anatomy and physiology related to all the following systems: cardiac; respiratory; neuro; endocrine; renal; musculoskeletal; gastro-intestinal; lymphatic;
- *immediate feedback*: MCQs normally employ automatic grading, therefore you can receive quick feedback and your result;
- *preparation*: due to the nature of MCQs being quick and easy to mark, your lecturers can provide you with the opportunity to have multiple formative attempts, which will support you in practising for the summative MCQ.

Succeeding in MCQs

Preparing to undertake an MCQ exam effectively involves a range of study techniques, some of which we will look at now.

- *Understand the content being assessed*:
    - review the module learning outcomes and be clear about the content being assessed; your lecturer will provide you with this information
    - review the modules' taught content and familiarise yourself with each area, covering the key concepts, theories and clinical knowledge required.

- *Practise with formative MCQs*:
    - your lecturer will provide opportunities for you to practise past MCQ papers
    - make sure you take this opportunity and practise as much as you can
    - use online databases or textbooks to help you practise – a lot of textbooks provide opportunities to undertake short MCQ tests.

- *Understand the structure of the question*:
    - be sure to understand what the question is asking – for example, does it say 'name', 'describe' and what are the key words, such as 'not', 'except', 'best', as this will help you focus on providing an accurate response
    - read all options carefully, and be mindful of trick answers – for example, the optional answers may all look the same apart from the use of key words.

- *Apply active recall and test your time management*:
    - test your own memory by trying to actively recall information without looking at your notes or textbook
    - practise undertaking an MCQ within the allocated time, and try not to focus on one question; if you are unsure of the answer, move to the next so you do not run out of time.

By using a range of study strategies, and regular practice, you can significantly improve your performance. Before moving on, let's look at some tips during the MCQ exam.

1. *Understand the question before you answer it*
    - read the question carefully – what is the question asking you to do? For example, does it say 'list' or does it say 'explain'?
    - look for the key words: for example, in 'give *two* examples', the key word here may be 'two'
    - look for trick answers – for example, you may be given three answers that seem the same, but when you read them carefully you might find only is one correct
    - look at the allocation of marks – some parts of the question may carry more marks, meaning a more comprehensive answer may be required.

2. *Remove wrong answers*
    - as you read the question, and answer, try to cross out the wrong answers first.

3. *Manage exam anxiety*
    - take a deep breath – you got this!
    - get plenty of rest the night before, and please try to eat breakfast
    - plan your journey to avoid rushing.

Now let's practise some MCQs.

Activity 8.2   Critical thinking

Now that you understand why MCQs are used in nurse education, use the following link to practise free online MCQs. This is just one resource; it would also be helpful at this stage for you to take time out and review your online module pages to see if your lecturer has released any further practice MCQ papers.

- Delves-Yates (2024) *Essentials of Nursing Practice: Multiple Choice Questions*. Available at: https://study.sagepub.com/essentialnursingpractice2e/student-resources/ace-your-assessment/multiple-chcice-questions

There is no model answer provided; the above link will also provide the answer to each of the MCQs.

Open- or closed-book exam

Traditionally, closed-book exams have been utilised in nurse education; however, the move to online teaching has increased the necessity to use open-book examinations. Like the MCQ, students often find undertaking a closed-book exam stressful, whereas open-book exams support students' confidence in undertaking assessments and can help decrease exam-related stress and anxiety. When comparing both types, lecturers believe that students invest more time and effort in preparing for closed-book exams, experiencing better outcomes. That being said, lecturers in favour of open-book exams believe that students can analyse and critique evidence from a variety of resources and, through the use of IT, can experience a deeper approach to learning (Johanns et al., 2017).

The decision to choose open- or closed-book exams will depend on what knowledge your lecturer is evaluating. Both sorts of exams have roles within nurse education, each with distinct advantages and disadvantages. The following sections aim to provide a comparison to help you in identifying the benefits and challenges with open- versus closed-book examinations.

Open-book exam

In an open-book exam, you can use your notes, textbooks and other resources such as articles, or websites while answering the exam questions.

Advantages

- *Less stress*: you may feel less pressure to retain and recall information, and you will feel less pressure knowing you can access materials to support you during the exam.
- *Reflects practice*: in clinical practice you will have access to a range of resources such as policies, guidelines and the internet to assist you in managing patient care. Therefore, using open-book exams can promote the use of authentic assessment as it reflects what you would or can do in practice.
- *Application of theory to practice*: open-book exams often work to test your ability to apply theory to practice using a range of resources, designed to assess your critical thinking and problem-solving skills.
- *Enhanced learning*: open-book exams are also a means to promote deeper learning, self-directed study and use of the supporting literature to underpin knowledge; therefore, they are seen as a teaching method as well as an assessment method.

Challenges

- *Time management*: open-book exams often have a time limit, so you will need to learn how to access the literature and reference quickly to ensure you do not run out of time.
- *Over-reliance*: often students can become over-reliant on the resources, and spend too much time looking up information as opposed to using their own knowledge.
- *Requires a deeper level of understanding*: using the resources alone will not suffice; you will need to show how you have used resources to demonstrate a deeper understanding of content being assessed. This is mainly why open-book exams are not normally used until the second or third year; first-year students are just beginning to learn and can't apply a deeper level of understanding in the same way.

Succeeding in open-book exams

- *Study*: an open-book exam can lead to students thinking they do not have to study – but you do need to. Remember, the open book acts to supplement your knowledge rather than answer the exam questions in their entirety.
- *Organisation*: organise your resources well – for example, use highlighters or sticky notes to mark items for quick reference.
- *Practise*: like MCQs, you must practise using an open book for examinations; use real-life scenarios and use a time limit. Time management and practice will be key in succeeding in open-book exams.

Closed-book exam

The alternative to an open-book exam is a closed-book exam, where you must rely on memory and recall; you are not permitted to view or use any source of information (Gamage et al., 2022).

Advantages

- *Academic integrity*: closed-book exams are less associated with cheating and therefore support students to apply academic integrity to their assessments.
- *Promote study*: they require you to prepare for the assessment, and promote the retention of knowledge and the ability to recall information.
- *Reflect practice*: closed-book exams test memory recall, therefore reflecting practice where nurses are expected to be able to recall information to deal with emergency situations in clinical practice.

Challenges

- *Stressful*: closed-book exams can be more stressful as you are expected to retain a lot of information.
- *Higher-order thinking*: this type of assessment tends to focus on measuring foundation knowledge and is useful in higher-order thinking.
- *Surface learning*: students tend to rote learn for closed-book assessments, which can be surface learning as opposed to deep understanding.

Succeeding in closed-book exams

- *Study*: preparation is key; avoid cramming before the exam as this can lead to stress and anxiety.
- *Active recall*: use flash cards, self-quizzing and previous exams to help you practise recalling information.

- *Practise*: review knowledge regularly to help you to reinforce memory and refrain from last-minute cramming of study.
- *Application to practice*: focus on applying knowledge to patient care as opposed to in isolation; this will help you recall information during the exam.

The above outlines the different approaches to written exams in nurse education, highlighting both similarities and differences, each with its own benefits and challenges. It is important to note that the layout of questions in exams may differ, with some using true/false, labelling of diagrams or short- and long-answer questions. The next section gives a brief overview of some of the different types of questions, but, prior to taking the exam, do ensure to confirm with your lecturer the type of questions that will be asked. This will help you prepare.

Types of questions within written exams

Whether undertaking an MCQ, open-book or closed-book exam, each will set out a variety of ways to test knowledge as follows.

- *Short-answer/essay questions*: used to test deeper understanding where you will be expected to give explanations, demonstrate problem-solving and use the literature to support your answers.
- *Case studies*: you will be given a detailed scenario, and may be asked to assess, plan and evaluate care of a patient, using the underpinning literature to support patient management. This approach is normally used to test your ability to apply theory to practice.
- *True or false questions*: used to assess your basic level of facts or concepts, and to check your knowledge related to principles of care – for example, normal blood pressure.
- *Fill-in-the-blank*: this approach will test your ability to recall specific terms, definitions or procedures related to patient care – for example, 'Tachycardic means fast ....'

Having looked at MCQs, open- and closed-book exams, use the next activity to test your understanding and application of what you have learned.

Activity 8.3   Reflection

Thinking about any recent exams you have undertaken, and using the information above, reflect on the following:

1. What were the advantages and challenges of the exam you sat?
2. How did you study for the exam, and what strategies helped you achieve a pass rate?

As this is a personal reflection, there is no model answer provided.

The final part of this chapter will focus on undertaking a drug calculation exam. This is a mandatory component within nurse education; it is a requirement to pass the course and qualify as an NMC registered nurse. Before this, let's have another look George's case study.

Case study: George, third-year student nurse, part 2

George is now in his third year of nursing. As part of the curriculum, he must undertake the drug calculation exam, where the pass mark is set at 100 per cent. George has been diligently preparing for this exam. He has attended all his classes, participated in study groups and completed numerous practice problems. Despite his efforts, he still wonders why the pass mark must be 100 per cent and whether he has practised enough to achieve this perfect score.

Activity 8.4　Reflection

Consider George's final case study.

1. Why is the pass mark 100 per cent?
2. Why is the drug calculation exam important?
3. How will George know he has prepared well for the exam?
4. What techniques could George use to reduce the stress associated with exams?
5. What are the common types of drug errors seen in practice?

A model answer is provided at the end of this chapter.

Drug calculation exam

Giving medications is one of the key responsibilities nurses take on; doing it safely means understanding pharmacology, how medications work and how to calculate the right doses. Throughout your training, you'll get plenty of hands-on experience with medication administration, both in class and during clinical placements. This mix of theory and practice will help you build the skills you need to give medications safely. Let's now take a look at what is meant by drug errors.

Drug errors

Drug errors occur 'either because of the numerical (mathematical) error, and/or because of the inability of the individual to conceptually extract the correct information from the drug calculation problem to set up the mathematical calculation needed' (McMullan et al., 2009, p. 892). A mathematical error relates to the incorrect ability to perform addition, subtraction, multiplication, division, or the use of decimals and fractions. Therefore, it is vital that you learn, practise and achieve proficiency in drug calculations during your nurse training. In addition to calculation errors, common medication administration mistakes are related to factors such as the patient, drug, dose, route and timing. This means that medication was given to the wrong patient, or the incorrect drug, dose or route of administration was used. Eaton (2023) stated that:

between April 2015 and March 2020 NHS Resolution received 1,420 claims relating to errors in the medication process (prescribing, preparing, dispensing, administering, monitoring or providing advice on medicines). Of the 1,420 claims received, 487 were settled at a cost to the NHS of £35 million.

This is an overwhelming record, and likely does not account for all errors; some may have gone unrecorded.

Drug calculation: pass mark

As previously mentioned, the NMC (2018) has outlined that calculation of medicines must be passed with a score of 100 per cent. This means that you need to be able to answer all drug calculations correctly. Minty-Walker et al. (2024) highlighted that the reason for the 100 per cent pass mark was to ensure public safety remained paramount. However, the high pass mark is what tends to cause the most stress among students, with students 'struggling to reach this expectation' and, ultimately, then failing their programme (Minty-Walker et al., 2024, p. 6). Your lecturers will provide numerous opportunities for you to practise and have drug calculation teaching sessions timetabled throughout your programme.

Most universities now have software such as SafeMedicate™ to help students practise drug calculations. SafeMedicate is an online platform designed to help students and healthcare professionals, particularly in nursing and medicine, enhance their medicine management skills. The platform focuses on improving patient safety and reducing medication errors by offering you interactive training modules and resources to support your continual learning. However, you will need to adopt strategies to help you succeed in drug calculations and utilise the resources provided to you throughout your programme to ensure you achieve the 100 per cent pass mark.

The next section will look at the drug calculation exam itself in more depth, highlighting some of the challenges students encounter and identifying strategies to help you succeed.

Layout of the drug calculation exam

- The exam will normally have ten questions to be completed in 30 minutes (25 per cent extra time permitted for students with a learning need, supported by the university).
- *100 per cent pass rate.*
- Variety of questions covering dosage calculations on patient weight or body surface area intravenous (IV) flow rates, concentration conversions – for example, milligram (mg) to microgram (mcg) – discussed in more detail below.
- Students undertaking nursing in children and young people will be questioned on paediatric dosages.
- Calculators are usually allowed as most students undertake the exam online at home, but make sure you check this with your lecturers first.

Types of calculations

- *Dosage calculations*: these relate to your ability to calculate the correct amount of a drug to administer based on the prescribed dosage.
- *IV flow rates*: calculating how fast an IV infusion should be administered.
- *Drug conversions*: you will be asked to convert between units of measurement, such as milligrams (mg) to grams (g), or millilitres (mL) to litres (L).
- *Weight-based*: this relates to your understanding of how to calculate the dosage of medications based on a patient's weight.

Exam format

- The drug calculations exam is normally presented in the format of MCQs/answers.
- The questions will reflect real-life medication scenarios to demonstrate your ability to apply theory to practice.
- The exam will be timed, which requires you to solve calculations under time pressure, reflecting the nature of clinical practice and time-sensitive patient-care situations.

Now let's look at the more common type of calculations you will undertake during the exam.

Oral medicines calculations

Brindley (2019) identified that the three areas of understanding needed to undertake the calculation of oral medications are as follows:

- conversion of units of measurement;
- formula for oral tablet/capsule calculations;
- formula for oral liquid preparations calculations.

The following three tables have been adapted from Brindley (2019) and will support you in the calculation of oral medicines.

Table 8.1   Conversion of units of measurement (adapted from Brindley, 2019, p. 2)

Unit sizes
• 1,000 nanograms (ng) = 1 microgram (mcg)
• 1,000mcg = 1 milligram (mg)
• 1,000mg = 1 gram (g)
Converting between measurements
• mcg to mg – you divide by 1,000
• mg to g – you divide by 1,000
• g to mg – you multiply by 1,000
• mg to mcg – you multiply by 1,000

Table 8.2   Formula for calculating oral tablets/capsules (adapted from Brindley, 2019, p. 2)

Formula
$\frac{What\ you\ want}{what\ you\ have}$ = What you give
• It is what you want (the dosage prescribed) divided by what you have (what dose of tablet do you have in stock) equals what you give in the dose prescribed.
Example
$\frac{40mg\ (the\ dose\ prescribed)}{10mg\ (dose\ in\ stock)}$ = 4 tablets (you need to give 4 x 10 mg tablets)

Table 8.3 Formula for calculating oral liquid preparations (adapted from Brindley, 2019, p. 2)

Formula

$\dfrac{\textit{What you want}}{\textit{what you have}} \times \textit{what is it in} = \textit{what you give}$

Example

For example, a patient has been prescribed 250mg erythromycin oral dose and is unable to take tablets or capsules. You have an oral suspension of

125mg erythromycin in 5mL

$\dfrac{250\text{mg}}{125\text{mg}} \times 5\text{mL} = \text{administer } 10\text{mL}$

Having reviewed some basic formulas for calculating oral and liquid medication and unit conversations, let's do some practice. The NMC has produced free practice tests which can help you check your understanding across 100s of drug calculations – we'll give it a try.

Activity 8.5   Critical thinking

Use the following link to access practice drug calculation test papers set out by the NMC. There are over 50 questions per paper, with 45 generic questions and five field-specific questions.
www.pearsonvue.com/us/en/nmc/practicetests.html

- access the above link;
- scroll to the bottom of the page;
- access 'Nursing' and you will see a list of papers to choose from.

There is no model answer to this as the answers are given within each of the practice papers.

Succeeding in drug calculation exams

The keys to succeeding in passing your drug calculation exam are, in part, as they are for any other exam. Some examples are as follows:

- *Understand basic maths skills*: learn to be comfortable using decimals, fractions and percentages, and utilise the formulas outlined previously in this chapter, including the conversion of units of measurements.
- *Focus on the common types of drug calculations*: your drug calculation exam will cover:
  o   oral
  o   liquid
  o   injectable medication
  o   IV infusions.

- Be clear on what else is required by speaking to your lecturer – for example, will you have generic and field-specific questions or just field-specific questions?
- *Practise*: the real trick to success with drug calculations is to take every opportunity to practise; do not leave it to the last minute. Use all the support your lecturers put in place – for example, maths sessions within teaching – and practise on previous exam papers. Also ensure you practise and can answer all questions within the allocated time, which is normally 30 minutes.
- *Check for common mistakes*: review the errors you are making. Some questions could be written in an ambiguous way to test reading comprehension and attention to detail; read the question carefully and make sure you understand what is being asked.
- *Stay calm*: during the exam it is important to stay calm (easy for me to say!); take a deep breath and focus on the task at hand. Allocate time for each question and, if you get stuck, move on to the next question and come back later. Don't rush and never guess; use note paper to work through calculations and use the calculator (if permitted).
- By practising and using the above steps, you will increase your confidence and ability to succeed in undertaking your drug calculation exam.

Conclusion

Written exams play a crucial role in assessing your knowledge and competency within nurse education. Exams are not only designed to evaluate your knowledge, but also act as assurance of your ability to work within ever-changing and complex clinical settings. This chapter discussed the various types of written exams, such as MCQs, short-answer questions and drug calculation exams, which are commonly used within nurse education. The chapter addressed the advantages and challenges with each format, alongside strategies that will help you succeed. A deeper look at drug calculation was undertaken within this chapter, and its links to the NMC. The consequences of medication administration errors were discussed, as well as a brief overview of basic conversion of units of measurement; the formulas for calculating oral tablet and oral liquid medications were provided. To aid you further this chapter has a number of embedded activities which will support your practice and study. By practising regularly, and understanding the relevance of the exam format, you will not only succeed in your written exams, but you will also ensure you are equipped to provide safe and effective care within the clinical settings, in line with the NMC requirements.

Brief outline answers

Activity 8.1 Reflection

1. How could George begin preparing for his upcoming MCQ exam?

He could begin with talking to his lecturer to discuss what is expected and to help understand the marking criteria. Looking at past exams papers is always a good idea; taking time to prepare and study will ensure George is successful on the day.

2. Who could George talk to about his concerns?

I would encourage George to speak with his peers, those who are in their second year; they will be able to offer some helpful insights into preparing for exams. George could also speak with the library support team at his university and his lecturers, who will be able to provide reassurance and offer support to help George prepare.

Activity 8.4 Reflection

1. Why is the pass mark 100 per cent?

This is set by the NMC to ensure students qualifying are equipped to safely administer medications.

2. Why is the drug calculation exam important?

It provides evidence that you have the necessary competence to safely calculate and administer medication.

3. How will George know he has prepared well for the exam?

If he is achieving the pass mark when using the practice exams he can feel confident that he has prepared and studied well before the exam.

4. What techniques could George use to reduce the stress associated with exams?

Breathe deeply; speak with his lecturers; use the recourses provided by his lecturers to prepare for the exam; study – do not cram; get a good night's sleep the night before; eat breakfast the morning of the exam; and make sure he maps out his journey (if the exam is at university as opposed to online).

5. What are the common types of drug errors seen in practice?

Using the incorrect unit of measurement and putting the decimal point in the wrong place. Often, errors are because the student has not taken the time to read the question before providing the answer.

Annotated further reading

Stunden, A. and Jefferies, D. (2018) The effectiveness of short answers test papers in evaluating academic nursing programs: a review of the literature. *Nurse Education Today*, 33, 94–101.

This is an interesting article that outlines the purpose and effectiveness of short-answer exams.

NMC (2021) *Practice Tests for the Test of Competence*. Available at: www.pearsonvue.com/us/en/nmc/practicetests.html

This website will give you access to lots of exam questions that relate to drug calculations.

References

Brindley, J. (2019) How to undertake oral medicines calculations. *Nursing Standard*, 34(7).

Delves-Yates, C. (2024) *Essentials of Nursing Practice: Multiple Choice Questions*. Available at: https://study.sagepub.com/essentialnursingpractice2e/student-resources/ace-your-assessment/multiple-choice-questions. Accessed 2 July 2025.

Eaton, D. (2023) Drug calculation skills for nurses. *Nursing Times*, September. Available at: www.nursingtimes.net/learning-units-and-portfolio/drug-calculation-skills-for-nurses-04-09-2023/. Accessed: 2 July 2025.

Gamage, K., Pradeep, R. and de Silva, E. (2022) Rethinking assessment: the future of examinations in higher education. *Sustainability*, 14, 3552.

Johanns, B., Dinkens, A. and Moore, J. (2017) A systematic review comparing open-book and closed-book examinations: evaluating effects on development of critical thinking skills. *Nurse Education in Practice*, 27, 89–94.

Leung, S., Mok, E. and Wong, D. (2008) The impact of assessment methods on the learning of nursing students. *Nurse Education Today*, 28, 711–19.

McMullan, M., Jones, R. and Lea, S. (2010) Patient safety: numerical skills and drug calculation abilities of nursing students and registered nurses. *Journal of Advanced Nursing*, 66, 891–9.

Minty-Walker, C., Wilson, N., Rylands, L., Pettigrew, J. and Hunt, L. (2024) Assessing numeracy and medication calculations within undergraduate nursing education: a qualitative study. *Nursing Open*, 11(7), 1–9.

NMC (2018) *Standards of Proficiency for Registered Nurses*. Available at: www.nmc.org.uk/globalassets/sitedocuments/standards/2024/standards-for-pre-registration-nursing-programmes.pdf. Accessed 2 July 2025.

Ortega-Sanchez, C. (2016) Written exams: how effectively are we using them? *Procedia: Social and Behavioural Sciences*, 228, 144–8.

Index

Index